A Guide to Migraine, Arthritis, Cervical Spondylosis and Backache

Published by
Lotus Press

A

Guide to

Migraine, Arthritis, Cervical Spondylosis and Backache

Dr. Rajeev Sharma

B.H.M.S; M.D. P.G.N.D; D.Y.Th., PMS

Lotus PRESS

4263/3, Ansari Road,

Darya Ganj, New Delhi-110002

Lotus Press
4263/3, Ansari Road, Darya Ganj,
New Delhi-110002 • Ph.: 32903912, 23280047
E-mail: lotus_press@sify.com • www.lotuspress.co.in

A Guide to Migraine, Arthritis,
Cervical Spondylosis and Backache

ISBN: 978-81-8382-253-4

Attention Readers:
Please consult to your physician before trying any medicine or treatment plan, Author/Publisher will not be responsible for any reaction/loss.

Published by: Lotus Press, New Delhi
Printed at: Anand Sons, Delhi

Preface

Headache/migraine, arthritis, backache etc. are very painful conditions of the body. Those who suffer from these disorders know the severity of symptoms and pain.

In this book, you will find about migraine, it's causes, types and prevention, cluster headache, mixed headache and headache in children etc. Besides headache, there is detailed description of arthritis, it's types and prevention. Backache is also covered in this book in a separate chapter.

This book contains description of proper exercises and yoga, which is supposed to be good supportive therapy for body pains. There are two separate chapters of homoeopathic treatment and a chapter on ayurvedic treatment too alongwith diet plan and home remedies.

If you want to come to my place, first fix an appointment and please do not come without appointment.

With thanks and regards,

Dr. Rajeev Sharma
E-mail: drs108@gmail.com

A Brief About

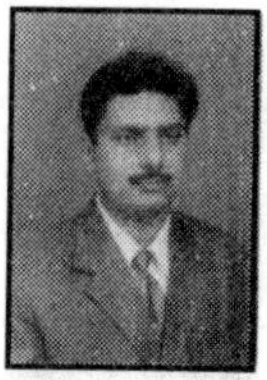

Dr. Rajeev Sharma is an eminent consultant of Homoeopathy,Yoga, Naturopathy and Alternative Medicine in India. He has written more than two hundred and fifty books (250) in Hindi and English and around one thousand articles which have been published in various newspapers and magazines. He was also an Editional Board Member of the prestigious *Asian Homoeopathic Journal* besides many other newspapers and magazines.

Dr. Rajeev Sharma has written books on ayurveda, allopathy, homoeopathy, yoga, naturopathy, accupressure, magnetotherapy, reiki, water-therapy, massage and aromatherapy etc.

The books written by Dr. Rajeev Sharma are published by renowned publishers of India. Besides this he is doing editing and translation also. He is content provider to many magazines.

Dr. Rajeev Sharma has written books on all major ailments like diabetes, hypertension, obesity, stomach and respiratory disorders, E.N.T. disorders, female disorders, UTI disorders, paediatric problems, headache, stress and other mental problems and Sexual Disorders etc. You can fix an appointment for any of such problem.

Dr. Rajeev Sharma is Medical Advisor to Ralson Remedies (a homoeopathic manufacturer), and Dixit Pharmacy (Ayurvedic Manufacturer), and Medical Officer in U.P. Govt.

He has received several prizes for his outstanding achievements. He has been awarded the *Best Author prize in Hindi* by the Ministry of Health and Family Welfare,

Government of India and *Sarjana Puraskar by U.P. Hindi Sansthan,* Lucknow. He has delivered talks on All India Radio and lectures on Alternative Medicine in various Government and Non-government Organisations. He has written Advt. Scripts for the products of several companies.

He is delivering lectures and providing literature on Yoga, Pranayama, Meditation, Stress and Life Style Management to the MNC's and corporate houses.

He has established a website through which you can get Online Training or e Books in Accupressure, Massage, Yoga, Water Therapy, Diet Therapy, Naturopathy, Colour Therapy and Reiki besides other paramedical courses.

Dr. Rajeev Sharma is also a social activist. He has worked a lot against Addiction and prevention of AIDS.

He has worked for human rights too and has received the World Human Rights Promotion Award. His name has been published in *LIMCA BOOK OF RECORDS* and is to be published in India Book of Records 2011.

He has developed a website :-
www.newkamasutra.com : A site of love, romance and sex.

Newkamasutra is a scientific site to guide for love, romance, relationship, dating, sex related and other problems. The information given here is not porn but scientific, relevant and authentic.You can update your knowledge by viewing "Vatsyayan's Kamasutra", "Newkamasutra", "Dating and Romance", "Sex Education", "Sexual Disorders", "Aphrodisiacs and Diets", "Sex Yoga" etc pages.

Besides this you can do "Consultation" and "Online Courses" or purchase an "eBook" of your choice or shop from "Store". "Forum" also provide facility to interact with viewers of our site.

We do not believe in magical remedies or untrue claims. We treat individuals on the basis of the totality of their symptoms. Thus the consultation and medicines provided are personalized.The ultimate aim of our organization is to provide quality information, medicines, teachings and techniques. This is called **QMT.**

Contents

1

Headache / Migraine

Oh my aching head! Nearly everyone has had a headache. The most common type of headache is a tension headache. Tension headaches are due to tight muscles in your shoulders, neck, scalp and jaw. They are often related to stress, depression or anxiety. You are more likely to get tension headaches if you work too much, don't get enough sleep, miss meals or use alcohol.

Other common types of headaches include migraines, cluster headaches and sinus headaches. Most people can feel much better by making lifestyle changes, learning ways to relax and taking pain relievers.

Headaches can have many causes, but serious causes of headaches are rare. Sometimes headaches warn of a more serious disorder. Let your health care provider know if you have sudden, severe headaches. Get medical help right away if you have a headache after a blow to your head, or if you have a headache along with a stiff neck, fever, confusion, loss of consciousness or pain in the eye or ear.

Migraine

A migraine is a common type of headache that may occur with symptoms such as nausea, vomiting, or sensitivity to light.

In many people, a throbbing pain is felt only on one side of the head.

Some people who get migraines have warning symptoms, called an aura, before the actual headache begins. An aura is a group of symptoms, usually vision disturbances, that serve as a warning sign that a bad headache is coming. Most people, however, do not have such warning signs.

Causes

A lot of people get migraines—about 11 out of 100. The headaches tend to first appear between the ages of 10 and 46. Occasionally, migraines may occur later in life in a person with no history of such headaches. Migraines occur more often in women than men, and may run in families. Women may have fewer migraines when they are pregnant. Most women with such headaches have fewer attacks during the last two trimesters of pregnancy.

A migraine is caused by abnormal brain activity, which is triggered by stress, certain foods, environmental factors, or something else. However, the exact chain of events remains unclear.

Scientists used to believe that migraines were due to changes in blood vessels within the brain. Today, most medical experts believe the attack actually begins in the brain itself, where it involves various nerve pathways and chemicals. The changes affect blood flow in the brain and surrounding tissues.

Migraine Attacks may be Triggered by:

- Alcohol
- Allergic reactions
- Bright lights
- Certain odours or perfumes

- Changes in hormone levels (which can occur during a woman's menstrual cycle or with the use of birth control pills)
- Changes in sleep patterns
- Exercise
- Loud noises
- Missed meals
- Physical or emotional stress
- Smoking or exposure to smoke

Certain foods and preservatives in foods may trigger migraines in some people. Food-related triggers may include:

- Any processed, fermented, pickled, or marinated foods
- Baked goods
- Chocolate
- Dairy products
- Foods containing monosodium glutamate (MSG)
- Foods containing tyramine, which includes red wine, aged cheese, smoked fish, chicken livers, figs, and certain beans
- Fruits (avocado, banana, citrus fruit)
- Meats containing nitrates (bacon, hot dogs, salami, cured meats)
- Nuts
- Onions
- Peanut butter

This List may not include all Triggers

True migraine headaches are not a result of a brain tumour or other serious medical problem. However, only an experienced health care provider can determine whether your symptoms are due to a migraine or another condition.

Symptoms

Vision disturbances, or aura, are considered a "warning sign" that a migraine is coming. The aura occurs in both eyes and may involve any or all of the following:

- A temporary blind spot
- Blurred vision
- Eye pain
- Seeing stars or zigzag lines
- Tunnel vision

Note: Every person with migraines has an aura. Those who do usually develop one about 10 - 15 minutes before the headache. However, it may occur just a few minutes to 24 hours beforehand. A headache may not always follow an aura.

Migraine headaches can be dull or severe. The pain may be felt behind the eye or in the back of the head and neck. For many patients, the headaches start on the same side each time. The headaches usually:

- feel throbbing, pounding, or pulsating
- are worse on one side of the head
- start as a dull ache and get worse within minutes to hours
- last 6 to 48 hours
- other symptoms that may occur with the headache include:
- Chills
- Increased urination
- Fatigue
- Loss of appetite
- Nausea and vomiting
- Numbness, tingling, or weakness
- Problems concentrating, trouble finding words
- Sensitivity to light or sound

- Sweating

Symptoms may linger even after the migraine has gone away. Patients with migraine sometimes call this a migraine "hangover." Symptoms can include:

- Feeling mentally dull, like your thinking is not clear or sharp
- Increased need for sleep
- Neck pain

Exams and Tests

Your doctor can diagnose this type of headache by asking questions about your symptoms and family history of migraines. A complete physical exam will be done to determine if your headaches are due to muscle tension, sinus problems, or a serious brain disorder.

There is no specific test to prove that your headache is actually a migraine. However, your doctor may order a brain MRI or CT scan if you have never had one before.

If you have a migraine with unusual symptoms such as weakness, memory problems, or loss of alertness, an EEG may be needed to rule out seizures. A lumbar puncture (spinal tap) might be done.

Treatment

There is no specific cure for migraine headaches. The goal is to prevent symptoms by avoiding or changing your triggers.

A good way to identify triggers is to keep a headache diary. Write down:

- When your headaches occur?
- How severe they are?
- What you've eaten?

- How much sleep you had?
- Other symptoms
- Other possible factors (women should note where they are in their menstrual cycle)

For example, the diary may reveal that your headaches tend to occur more often on days when you wake up earlier than usual. Changing your sleep schedule may result in fewer migraine attacks.

When you do get migraine symptoms, try to treat them right away. The headache may be less severe. When migraine symptoms begin:

- Drink water to avoid dehydration, especially if you have vomited
- Rest in a quiet, darkened room
- Place a cool cloth on your head

Many different medications are available for people with migraines. Medicines are used to:

- reduce the number of attacks
- stop the migraine once early symptoms occur
- treat the pain and other symptoms

Reducing Attacks

If you have frequent migraines, your doctor may prescribe medicine to reduce the number of attacks. Such medicine needs to be taken every day in order to be effective. Such medications may include:

- Antidepressants such as amitriptyline
- Blood pressure medicines such as beta blockers (propanolol) or calcium channel blockers (verapamil)
- Seizure medication such as valproic acid, gabepentin, and topiramate

- Serotonin reuptake inhibitors (SSRIs) such as venlafaxine
- Selective norepinephrine uptake inhibitor (SNRIs) such as duloxetine

Stopping an Attack

Other medicines are taken at the first sign of a migraine attack. Over-the-counter pain medications such as acetaminophen, ibuprofen, or aspirin are often helpful, especially when your migraine is mild. If these don't help, ask your doctor about prescription medications. (Be aware, however, that overuse or misuse of such pain medications may result in rebound headaches.Chronic rebound headaches typically occur in people who take pain medications more than 3 days a week on an ongoing basis.)

Your doctor can select from several different types of medications, including:

- Triptans—the most frequently prescribed medicines for stopping migraine attacks—such as almotriptan (Axert), frovatriptan (Frova), rizatriptan (Maxalt), sumatriptan (Imitrex), and zolmitriptan (Zomig)
- Ergots such as dihydroergotamine or ergotamine with caffeine (Cafergot)
- Isometheptene (Midrin)

These medications come in different forms. Patients who have nausea and vomiting with their migraines may be prescribed a nasal spray, suppository, or injection instead of pills.

Some migraine medicines narrow your blood vessels and should not be used if you are at risk for heart attacks or have heart disease, unless otherwise instructed by your health care provider. Ergots should not be taken if you are pregnant or planning to become pregnant, because they can cause serious side effects to an unborn baby.

Carotidynia, also called lower-half headache or facial migraine, produces deep, dull, aching, and sometimes piercing pain in the jaw or neck. There is usually tenderness and swelling over the carotid artery in the neck. Episodes can occur several times weekly and last a few minutes to hours. This type occurs more commonly in older people. Doppler ultrasound studies of the carotid arteries are normal.

Headache-free migraine is characterized by the presence of aura without headache. This occurs in patients with a history of migraine with aura.

Ophthalmoplegic migraine begins with a headache felt in the eye and is accompanied by vomiting. As the headache progresses, the eyelid droops (ptosis) and nerves responsible for eye movement become paralyzed. Ptosis may persist for days or weeks.

Status migraine is a rare type involving intense pain that usually lasts longer than 72 hours. The patient may require hospitalization.

Incidence and Prevalence

Migraines afflict about 30 million people in the United States. They may occur at any age, but usually begin between the ages of 10 and 40 and diminish after age 50. Some people experience several migraines a month, while others have only a few migraines throughout their lifetime. Approximately 75% of migraine sufferers are women.

Prevention

Understanding your headache triggers can help you avoid foods and situations that cause your migraines. Keep a headache diary to help identify the source or trigger of your symptoms. Then modify your environment or habits to avoid future headaches.

Other tips for preventing migraines include:

- Avoid smoking
- Avoid alcohol
- Avoid artificial sweeteners and other known food-related triggers
- Get regular exercise
- Get plenty of sleep each night

Exams and Tests

Your health care provider can diagnosis this type of headache by performing a physical exam and asking questions about your symptoms and medical history.

If a physical exam is done during an attack, the exam will usually reveal Horner syndrome (one-sided eyelid drooping or a small pupil). These symptoms will not be present at other times. No other neurological changes will be seen.

Tests, such as an MRI of the head, may be needed to rule out other causes for the headaches.

Treatment

Treatment does not cure cluster headaches. The goal of treatment is to relieve symptoms. The headaches may go away on their own, or you may need treatment to prevent them.

Smoking, alcohol use, specific foods, and other factors that seem to trigger cluster headaches should be avoided. A headache diary can help you identify your headache triggers. When you get a headache, write down the day and time the pain began. The diary should include notes about what you ate and drank in the last 24 hours, how much you slept and when, and what was going on in your life immediately before the pain started. For example, were you under any unusual stress? Also include information about how long the headache lasted, and what made it stop.

Treatment for cluster headaches involves:

- Methods to treat the pain when it happens
- Medicines to prevent the headaches

Your doctor may recommend the following treatments when the headaches occur

- Triptans, such as sumatriptan (Imitrex)

- Several weeks of anti-inflammatory (steroid) medicines such as prednisone — starting with a high dose, then gradually decreased
- Breathing in 100% (pure) oxygen, often relieves cluster headache for some people, particularly for frequent cluster headaches that occur at night
- Injections of the drug known as dihydroergotamine (DHE), which can stop cluster attacks within 5 minute (Warning: this drug can be dangerous if taken with sumatriptan)

A combination of medicines may be needed to control headache symptoms. Because each person responds differently to medicine, your doctor may have you try several medications before deciding which works best for you.

Painkillers do not usually relieve the pain from cluster headaches. Generally, they take too long to work.

The following medications may also be used to treat or prevent headache symptoms:

- Antiseizure medications such as topiramate and valproic acid
- Indomethacin or naproxen
- Lithium carbonate
- Calcium channel blockers such as verapamil
- Propranolol
- Amitriptyline
- Cyproheptadine

In rare cases, surgery on certain nerve cells near the brain may be recommended if medications do not work.

Outlook (Prognosis)

Cluster headaches are not life-threatening and usually cause no permanent structural changes. However, they are chronic

3

Mixed Tension Migraine

Symptoms

- Headache on one or both sides
    - o Throbbing pain
    - o May feel dull, tight, or like a band around the head
    - o Pain varies from mild to severe
    - o May get worse with activity
    - o May last 4 - 72 hours (in some people, the headaches may occur every day)
- Nausea or vomiting
- Sensitivity to light or sound
- Irritability
- Depression
- Sluggishness
- Numbness, tingling, weakness
- Neck pain

Exams and Tests

Your doctor will perform a physical exam, including a detailed examination of your nervous system, and ask you about your symptoms and family history.

Tests that may be done include:

- CT or MRI of the head and neck
- Blood work
- Lumbar puncture (spinal tap)

Treatment

Certain things may cause your headaches. For example, some people get headaches after drinking alcohol or eating certain foods. These are called triggers. You should identify your specific triggers and avoid them as much as possible.

A headache diary can help you identify your headache triggers. When you get a headache, write down the day and time the pain began. The diary should include notes about what you ate and drank in the last 24 hours, how much you slept and when, and what was going on in your life immediately before the pain started. For example, were you under any unusual stress? Also include information about how long the headache lasted, and what made it stop.

Hot or cold showers or baths may relieve a headache for some people. It is important to follow a healthy lifestyle, get plenty of sleep, and to avoid stress as much as possible.

Over-the-counter medicines such as ibuprofen and acetaminophen may help. If your headaches are severe, your doctor may prescribe other medicines to relieve your pain and prevent further attacks.

Outlook (Prognosis)

Avoiding triggers and taking the appropriate medicine can help manage headache symptoms in many people.

Possible Complications

Pain medications only relieve headache symptoms for a short period of time. After a while, they do not work as well or the help they provide does not last as long. Regular, overuse of pain medications can lead to rebound headaches. Typically this occurs in people who take pain medications 3 or more times a week on a regular basis.

It's important to see a doctor if you have chronic headaches. In some cases, the headache may be a symptom of a more serious disorder.

sleeping with the neck in an abnormal position may also trigger a tension headache.

Other triggers of tension headaches include:

- Alcohol use
- Caffeine (too much or withdrawal)
- Colds and flu
- Dental problems such as jaw clenching or teeth grinding
- Eye strain
- Excessive smoking
- Fatigue
- Nasal congestion
- Over exertion
- Sinus infection

Tension headaches are not associated with structural changes in the brain.

Symptoms

The headache pain may be described as:

- Dull, pressure-like (not throbbing)
- A tight band or vise on the head
- All over (not just in one point or one side)
- Worse in the scalp, temples, or back of the neck, and possibly in the shoulders

The pain may occur as an insolated event, constantly, or daily. Pain may last for 30 minutes to 7 days. It may be triggered by or get worse with stress, fatigue, noise, or glare.

There may be difficulty in sleeping. Tension headaches usually do not cause nausea or vomiting.

People with tension headaches tend to try relieve pain by massaging their scalp, temples, or the bottom of the neck.

Exams and Tests

A headache that is mild to moderate, not accompanied by other symptoms, and responds to home treatment within a few hours may not need further examination or testing, especially if it has occurred in the past. A tension headache reveals no abnormal findings on a neurological exam. However, tender points (trigger points) in the muscles are often seen in the neck and shoulder areas.

The health care provider should be consulted — to rule out other disorders that can cause headache — if the headache is severe, persistent (does not go away), or if other symptoms are present with the headache.

Headaches that disturb sleep, occur whenever you are active, or that are recurrent or chronic may require examination and treatment by a health care provider.

Treatment

Understanding your headache triggers can help you avoid situations that cause your headaches. A headache diary can help you identify your headache triggers. When you get a headache, write down the day and time the pain began. The diary should include notes about what you ate and drank in the last 24 hours, how much you slept and when, and what was going on in your life immediately before the pain started. For example, were you under any unusual stress? Also include information about how long the headache lasted, and what made it stop.

Hot or cold showers or baths may relieve a headache for some people. You may need to make lifestyle changes if you have chronic tension headaches. This may include changing your sleep habits (usually to get more sleep), increasing exercise, and stretching the neck and back muscles. In some situations, you may need to change your job or recreational habits.

Over-the-counter painkillers such as aspirin, ibuprofen, or acetaminophen may relieve pain if relaxation techniques do not work. If you are planning to take part in an activity that you know will trigger a headache, taking one of these painkillers beforehand may be helpful.

Narcotic pain relievers are sometimes prescribed. Remember that pain medications only relieve headache symptoms for a short period of time. After a while, they do not work as well or the help they provide does not last as long. Regular, overuse of pain medications can lead to rebound headaches.

Other prescription treatments may include:

- Muscle relaxants such as tizanidine
- Selective serotonin-reuptake inhibitors (SSRIs) such as paroxetine (Paxil) or citalopram (Celexa) taken daily to help prevent or decrease the number of headaches
- Tricyclic antidepressants such as amitriptyline, nortriptyline, or doxepin taken daily to help prevent or decrease the number of headaches

Combining drug treatment with relaxation or stress-management training, biofeedback, cognitive behavioural therapy, or acupuncture may provide better relief for chronic headaches.

Botox (botulinum toxin) is becoming popular as a treatment for chronic daily headaches, including tension headaches. However, it is currently not approved for such use.

Outlook (Prognosis)

Tension headaches usually respond well to treatment without residual effects.

Although they are not medically dangerous, chronic tension headaches can have a negative impact on the quality of life and work productivity.

Possible Complications

Rebound headaches — headaches that keep coming back — may occur from overuse of painkillers.

It's important to see a doctor if you have chronic headaches. In some cases, the headache may be a symptom of a more serious disorder.

Prevention

Learn and practice stress management. Some people find relaxation exercises or meditation helpful. Biofeedback may improve relaxation exercises and may be helpful for chronic tension headache.

Tips to prevent tension headaches:

- Keep warm if the headache is associated with cold.
- Use a different pillow or change sleeping positions.
- Practice good posture when reading, working, or doing other activities.
- Exercise the neck and shoulders frequently when typing, working on computers, or doing other close work.
- Get plenty of sleep and rest.

Massaging sore muscles may also help.

• • •

5

Stress Management

Stress is a feeling of emotional or physical tension.

Information

Emotional stress usually occurs in situations people consider difficult or challenging. Different people consider different situations to be stressful.

Physical stress refers to a physical reaction of the body to various triggers. The pain experienced after surgery is an example of physical stress. Physical stress often leads to emotional stress, and emotional stress often occurs as physical stress (e.g., stomach cramps).

Stress management involves controlling and reducing the tension that occurs in stressful situations by making emotional and physical changes. The degree of stress and the desire to make the changes will determine how much change takes place.

Assessing Stress

Attitude: A person's attitude can influence whether or not a situation or emotion is stressful. A person with a negative attitude will often report more stress than would someone with a positive attitude.

Diet: A poor diet puts the body in a state of physical stress and weakens the immune system. As a result, a person can be more likely to get infections. A poor diet can mean unhealthy food choices, not eating enough, or not eating on a normal schedule.

This form of physical stress also decreases the ability to deal with emotional stress, because not getting the right nutrition may affect the way the brain processes information.

Physical activity: Not getting enough physical activity can put the body in a stressed state. Physical activity has many benefits, including promoting a feeling of well-being.

Support systems: Almost everyone needs someone in their life they can rely on when they are having a hard time. Having little or no support makes stressful situations even more difficult to deal with.

Relaxation: People with no outside interests, hobbies, or other ways to relax may be less able to handle stressful situations.

- Find the positive in situations, and don't dwell on the negative.
- Plan fun activities
- Take regular breaks.

Physical Activity:

- Start a physical activity program. Most experts recommend 20 minutes of aerobic activity three times per week.
- Decide on a specific type, amount, and level of physical activity. Fit this into your schedule so it can be part of your routine.
- Find a buddy to exercise with — it is more fun and it will encourage you to stick with your routine.
- You do not have to join a gym — 20 minutes of brisk walking outdoors is enough.

Nutrition:

- Eat foods that improve your health and well-being. For example, increase the amount of fruits and vegetables you eat.
- Use the food guide pyramid to help you make healthy food choices.
- Eat normal-sized portions on a regular schedule.

Social Support:

- Make an effort to socialize. Even though you may feel tempted to avoid people when you feel stressed, meeting friends usually helps people feel less stressed.
- Be good to yourself and others.

Relaxation:

- Learn about and try using relaxation techniques, such as guided imagery, listening to music, or practicing yoga or meditation. With some practice, these techniques should work for you.
- Listen to your body when it tells you to slow down or take a break.
- Make sure to get enough sleep. Good sleep habits are one of the best ways to manage stress.
- Take time for personal interests and hobbies.

Resources

If these stress management techniques do not work for you, there are professionals, such as licensed social workers, psychologists, and psychiatrists, who can help. Schedule time with one of these mental health professionals to help you learn stress management strategies, including relaxation techniques. Support groups of various types are also available in most communities.

• • •

6

Headache in Children and Sleep Disorder

Children and Headache

Headaches are common in children. Headaches that begin early in life can develop into migraines as the child grows older. Migraines in children or adolescents can develop into tension-type headaches at any time. In contrast to adults with migraine, young children often feel migraine pain on both sides of the head and have headaches that usually last less than 2 hours. Children may look pale and appear restless or irritable before and during an attack. Other children may become nauseous, lose their appetite, or feel pain elsewhere in the body during the headache.

Headaches in children can be caused by a number of triggers, including emotional problems such as tension between family members, stress from school activities, weather changes, irregular eating and sleep, dehydration, and certain foods and drinks. Of special concern among children are headaches that occur after head injury or those accompanied by rash, fever, or sleepiness.

It may be difficult to identify the type of headache because children often have problems describing where it hurts, how often the headaches occur, and how long they last. Asking a child with a headache to draw a picture of where the pain is and how it feels can make it easier for the doctor to determine the proper treatment.

Migraine in particular is often misdiagnosed in children. Parents and caretakers sometimes have to be detectives to help determine that a child has migraine. Clues to watch for include sensitivity to light and noise, which may be suspected when a child refuses to watch television or use the computer, or when the child stops playing to lie down in a dark room. Observe whether or not a child is able to eat during a headache. Very young children may seem cranky or irritable and complain of abdominal pain (abdominal migraine).

Headache treatment in children and teens usually includes rest, fluids, and over-the-counter pain relief medicines. Always consult with a physician before giving headache medicines to a child. Most tension-type headaches in children can be treated with over-the-counter medicines that are marked for children with usage guidelines based on the child's age and weight. Headaches in some children may also be treated effectively using relaxation/behavioural therapy. Children with cluster headache may be treated with oxygen therapy early in the initial phase of the attacks.

Headache and Sleep Disorders

Headaches are often a secondary symptom of a sleep disorder. For example, tension-type headache is regularly seen in persons with insomnia or sleep-wake cycle disorders. Nearly three-fourths of individuals who suffer from narcolepsy complain of either migraine or cluster headache. Migraines and cluster headaches appear to be related to the number of and transition between rapid eye movement (REM) and other sleep periods an individual has during sleep. Hypnic headache awakens individuals mainly at night but may also interrupt daytime naps. Reduced oxygen levels in people with sleep apnea may trigger early morning headaches.

Getting the proper amount of sleep can ease headache pain. Generally, too little or too much sleep can worsen headaches, as can overuse of sleep medicines. Daytime naps often reduce deep sleep at night and can produce headaches in some adults. Some sleep disorders and secondary headache are treated using antidepressants. Check with a doctor before using over-the-counter medicines to ease sleep-associated headaches.

• • •

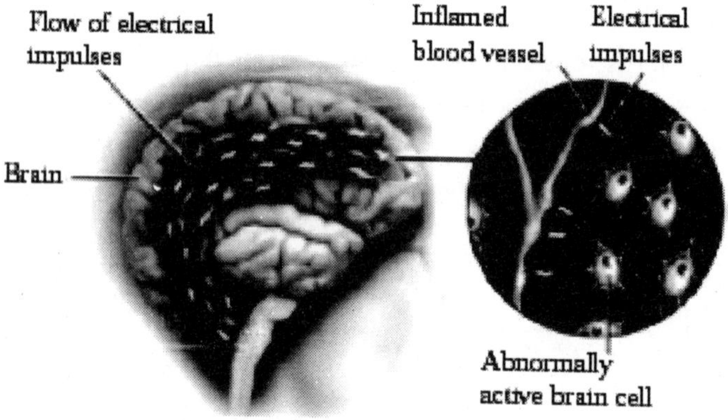

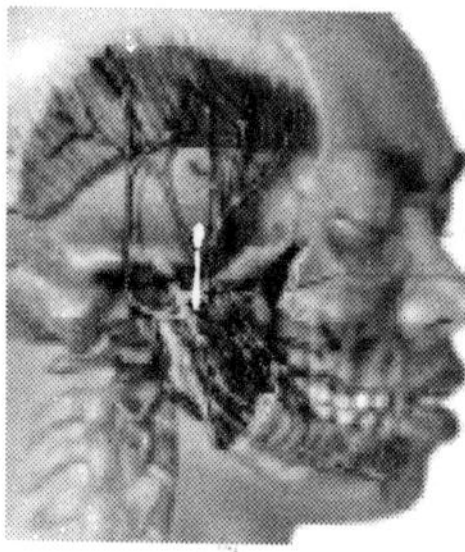

Nerves branching of the brainstem may become overexcited leading to dilatation of blood vessels

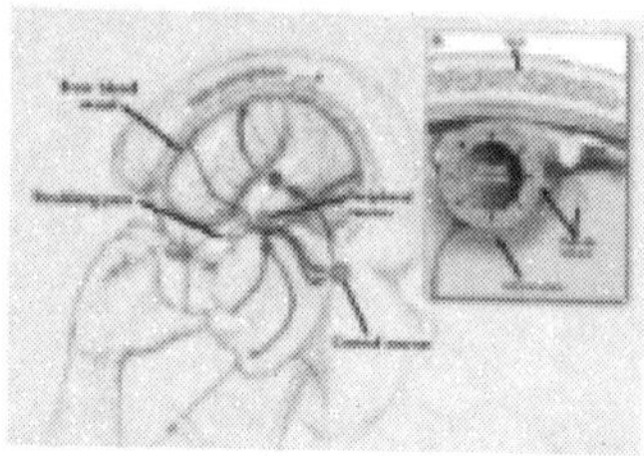

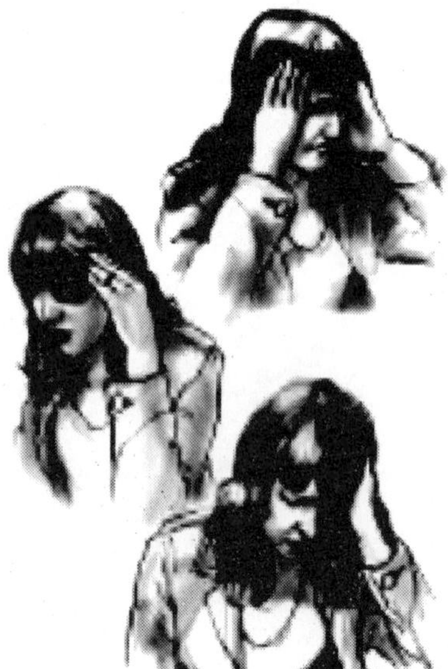

7

Arthritis–Causes and Symptoms

Did you know that there are more than 100 types of arthritis? Common arthritis symptoms of inflammation, pain, and stiffness are usually caused by degenerative arthritis (osteoarthritis). Other types of arthritis include rheumatoid arthritis and gout.Rheumatoid arthritis is a painful disease that can destroy joints. Women are three times more likely to get it than men.

What is Arthritis?

The word "arthritis" means "joint inflammation." Inflammation is one of the body's natural reactions to disease or injury, and includes swelling, pain, and stiffness. Inflammation that lasts for a very long time or recurs, as in arthritis, can lead to tissue damage.

A joint is where two or more bones come together, such as the hip or knee. The bones of a joint are covered with a smooth, spongy material called cartilage, which cushions the bones and allows the joint to move without pain. The joint is lined by a thin film of tissue called the synovium. The synovium's lining produces a slippery fluid called synovial fluid that nourishes the joint and helps reduce friction. Strong bands of tissue, called ligaments, connect the bones and help keep the joint stable. Muscles and tendons also support the joints and enable you to move.

With arthritis, an area in or around a joint becomes inflamed, causing pain, stiffness and, sometimes, difficulty moving. Some types of arthritis also affect other parts of the body, such as the skin and internal organs.

Rheumatoid Arthritis Linked to Sunshine Vitamin Deficiency

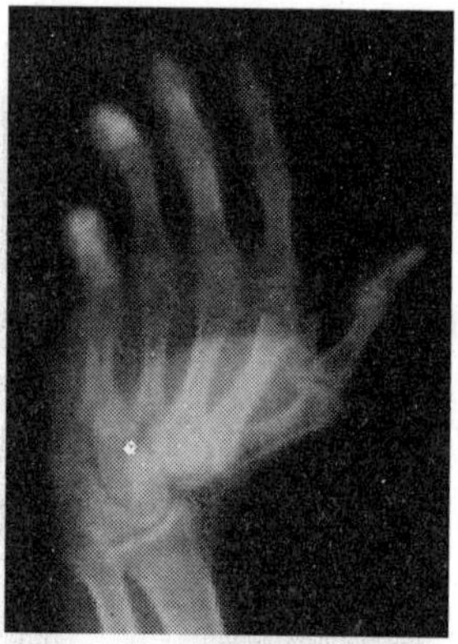

Researchers from the Boston University School of Public Health, Boston, United States, established a significant relationship between vitamin D and the risk for rheumatoid arthritis by observing women living in north-eastern America, who were found to be more likely to develop rheumatoid arthritis.

Details of Study

The researchers said that there is a definitive link between the vitamin D deficiency and RA risk as they found that women living in more northern latitudes showed a higher prevalence of rheumatoid arthritis as they had lower levels of sunshine vitamin due to less exposure to sunlight.

For the study, scientists looked at the data collected from the Nurses' Health Study, observing the facts such as behavioural risk factors, health outcomes and residential addresses of subjects between 1988 and 2002.

They based their results on 461 women who had rheumatoid arthritis, as compared to a large control group of 9,220 females.

The authors wrote, "A geographic association with northern latitudes has also been observed for multiple sclerosis and Crohn's disease, other autoimmune diseases that may be mediated by reduced vitamin D from decreased solar exposure and the immune effects of vitamin D deficiency."

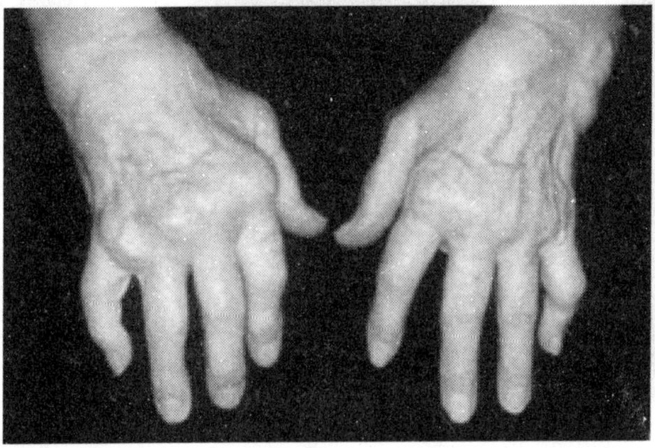

Facts about Vitamin D

It is found in fish like salmon, egg yolks and margarine.

Medical studies have suggested that Vitamin D may also help with seasonal affective disorder (SAD).

As little as 30 minutes of early morning or late afternoon sunlight on the face, hands and arms two or three times a week can supply the entire Vitamin D one needs.

Types of Arthritis

There are more than 100 different types of arthritis. Some of the more common types include:

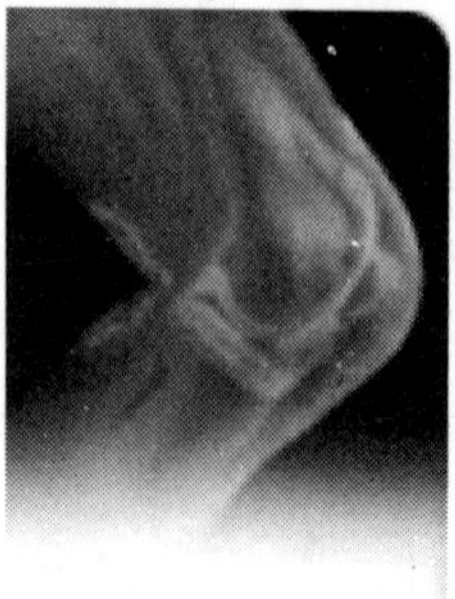

- **Osteoarthritis:** This is the most common type of arthritis. It occurs when the cartilage covering the end of the bones gradually wears away. Without the protection of the cartilage, the bones begin to rub against each other and the resulting friction leads to pain and swelling. Osteoarthritis can occur in any joint, but most often affects the hands and weight-bearing joints such as the knee, hip and facet joints (in the spine). Osteoarthritis often occurs as the cartilage breaks down, or degenerates, with age or overuse. For this reason, osteoarthritis is sometimes called degenerative joint disease.
- **Rheumatoid arthritis:** Rheumatoid arthritis is a long-lasting disease that can affect joints in any part of the body except the lower back and most commonly involves the hands, wrists, and knees. With rheumatoid arthritis, the immune system — the body's defense system against disease — mistakenly attacks itself and causes the joint lining to swell. The inflammation then spreads to the surrounding tissues, and can eventually damage cartilage and bone. In more severe cases, rheumatoid arthritis can affect other areas of the body, such as the skin, eyes, lungs, and nerves.
- **Gout:** Gout is a painful condition that occurs when the body cannot eliminate a natural substance called uric acid. The excess uric acid forms needle-like crystals in the joints

that cause swelling and severe pain. Gout most often affects the big toe, knee, and wrist joints.

Inaccurate Information about Arthritis Persists and is often Spread

- Arthritis is an old person's disease.
- Arthritis is induced by a cold, wet climate; (may be but not always).
- Arthritis can be cured.
- Arthritis is caused by a poor diet.
- Arthritis consists of only minor aches and pains.
- "You felt fine yesterday....why so tired today?"

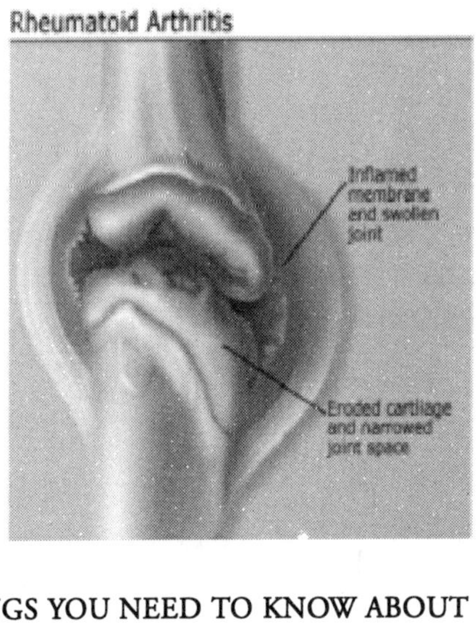

Eight things you need to know about Rheumatoid Arthritis

1. It's a lifelong condition.
2. It's not an 'older person's disease'.People can develop it at any age, even as children. For most people symptoms generally begin between 40 and 60 years of age.

3. There is no obvious pattern to the symptoms. Everybody's disease is different. People get 'flares', or periods when their symptoms are much worse, which then subside.You can have periods when the disease is quiet and doesn't cause you any problems.
4. It doesn't only affect the joints.It can sometimes affect other parts of the body, for example the eyes and lungs, though not for everyone.Apart from joint pain, stiffness and swelling, some people may have difficulty in sleeping, feel intensely tired and feel like they have bad flu.
5. It's a type of disease called an 'autoimmune disease', which results from a problem with the body's immune system.
6. Left untreated, it is a destructive disease that can cause serious damage to joints, if the inflammation is not controlled.
7. Some people have very little damage to their joints and a few (about 1 in 20) have severe damage in several joints. It is a progressive disease, but how it progresses varies from person to person. Treatment aims to control the disease and reduce the damage.
8. With early diagnosis and the right treatment, most people diagnosed today can expect to lead normal lives with their symptoms under control.

Exercises

Try to **keep active**, even if you don't always feel like it. It's about finding a balance between getting enough rest,and being active enough to keep your muscles strong and your joints mobile without harming them. Swimming can be ideal, because the joints are supported while you exercise. And you don't have to pay for exercise for it to do you good – walking counts!

Gentle stretching exercises help to keep you mobile. Making small changes to your daily routine now will add up over time so that you feel the benefits.

What Are the Symptoms of Arthritis?

Different types of arthritis have different symptoms and the symptoms vary in severity from person to person. Osteoarthritis does not generally cause any symptoms outside the joint. Symptoms of other types of arthritis may include fatigue, fever, a rash, and the signs of joint inflammation, including:

- Pain
- Swelling
- Stiffness
- Tenderness
- Redness
- Warmth

What is Rheumatoid Factor?

Rheumatoid factor is an immunoglobulin (antibody) which can bind to other antibodies. Antibodies are normal proteins found in the blood which function within the immune system. Rheumatoid factor though is not normally found in the general population (only found in about 1-2% of healthy people). The incidence of rheumatoid factor increases with age and about 20% of people over 65 years old have an elevated rheumatoid factor.

A blood test is used to detect the presence of rheumatoid factor. The blood test is commonly ordered to diagnose rheumatoid arthritis. Rheumatoid factor is present in 80% of adults who have rheumatoid arthritis but there is a much lower prevalence in juvenile rheumatoid arthritis.

Other Conditions Can Test Positive For Rheumatoid Factor

Other autoimmune diseases can also be positive for rheumatoid factor including:

- Sjogren's syndrome
- Systemic lupus erythematosus
- Scleroderma
- Polymyositis
- Dermatomyositis
- Mixed Connective Tissue Disease

Other infections or conditions which can be associated with positive rheumatoid factor include:

- Bacterial endocarditis
- Osteomyelitis
- Tuberculosis
- Syphilis
- Hepatitis
- Mononucleosis
- Diffuse interstitial pulmonary fibrosis
- Liver cirrhosis
- Sarcoidosis

Conditions Not Associated With Rheumatoid Factor

Rheumatic conditions NOT associated with elevated rheumatoid factor include:

- Osteoarthritis
- Ankylosing spondylitis
- Gout
- Psoriatic arthritis
- Reiter's syndrome / Reactive arthritis

High levels or titers of rheumatoid factor are associated with more severe rheumatoid arthritis. The factor also has been associated with a higher tendency to develop the non-joint complications of the disease such as rheumatoid nodules and rheumatoid lung disease.

Indicated Homoeopathic Medicines

Acid formic

- Chronic Myalgia, Gout and articular rheumatism, Acute rheumatic fever
- Pains worse on right side, motion, Better from motion

Colchicum

- The parts are red, hot, swollen, Tearing pains, worse in the evening, at night and from touch
- Feeling of pins and needles in hands and wrists, Finger tips are numb
- Inflammation of great toe, Gout in the heel, cannot bear to have it touched or moved

Dulcamara

- Rheumatic problems induced by damp cold, relieved by moving about
- Paralysis of single parts, Feet icy cold
- Rheumatic symptoms after acute skin eruption

Gelsemium

- Lac of muscular coordination, Sluggish circulation
- Excessive trembling and weakness of all the limbs
- Worse by damp weather, fog, thunderstorm, excitement, bad news, tobacco smoking, thinking of ailments, Better by bending forward, profuse micturition, open air, continuous motion.

Ledum Pal

- Gouty pains shoot all through the foot and limb, especially joints
- Gouty nodosities, Ball of great toe swollen
- Rheumatism begins in lower limbs and ascends, worse warmth of bed

Lithium Carb

- Chronic rheumatism connected with heart lesions
- Uric acid diathesis, Nodular swellings in joints, Better hot water.
- Rheumatic pains throughout shoulder joint, arm, fingers and small joints

Natrum Salicylicum

- Acute articular rheumatism and Lumbago

Rhus Tox

- Rheumatism in the cold season, Hot, painful swelling of joints
- Rheumatic pains spread over a large surface at nape of neck, back and extremities
- Better by motion, The cold fresh air is not tolerated

Homoeopathic manufacturer Ralson Remedies has prepared a patent named RALRHEUMO, which has all these ingredients.

• • •

8

Arthritis Pain and It's Relief

The pain of arthritis may come from different sources. These may include inflammation of the synovial membrane (tissue that lines the joints), the tendons, or the ligaments; muscle strain; and fatigue. A combination of these factors contributes to the intensity of the pain.

The pain of arthritis varies greatly from person to person, for reasons that doctors do not yet understand completely. Factors that contribute to the pain include swelling within the joint, the amount of heat or redness present, or damage that has occurred within the joint. In addition, activities affect pain differently so that some patients not pain in their joints after first getting out of bed in the morning whereas others develop pain after prolonged use of the joint. Each individual has a different threshold and tolerance for pain, often affected by both physical and emotional factors. These can include depression, anxiety, and even hypersensitivity at the affected sites due to inflammation and tissue injury. This increased sensitivity appears to affect the amount of pain perceived by the individual.

Measuring Arthritis Pain?

Pain is a private, unique experience that cannot be seen. The most common way to measure pain is for the doctor to ask you, the patient, about your problems. For example, the doctor may ask you to describe the level of pain you feel on a scale of 1 to 10. You may use words like aching, burning, stinging, or throbbing. These words will give the doctor a clearer picture of the pain you are experiencing. Since doctors rely on your description of pain to help guide treatment, you may want to keep a pain diary to record your pain sensations. On a daily basis, you can describe the situations that cause or alter the intensity of your pain, the sensations and severity of your pain, and your reactions to the pain. For example:

"On Sunday night, sharp pains in my knees produced by housework interfered with my sleep; on Monday morning, because of the pain, I had a hard time getting out bed. However, I coped with the pain by taking my medication and applying ice to my knees."

The diary will give the doctor some insight into your pain and may play a critical role in the management of your disease.

What will Happen when You First Visit a Doctor for your Arthritis Pain?

- Take your medical history and ask questions such as: How long have you had this problem? How intense is the pain? How often does it occur? What causes it to get worse? What causes it to get better?
- Review the medications you are using
- Conduct a physical examination
- Take blood and/or urine samples and request necessary laboratory work
- Ask you to get X-rays taken or undergo other imaging procedures such as a CAT scan (computerized axial tomography) or MRI (magnetic resonance imaging).

Once the doctor has done these things and reviewed the results of any tests or procedures, he or she will discuss the findings with you and design a comprehensive management approach for the pain caused by your osteoarthritis or rheumatoid arthritis.

Who Can Treat Arthritis Pain?

A number of different specialists may be involved in the care of an arthritis patient often a team approach is used. The team may include doctors who treat people with arthritis (rheumatologists), surgeons (orthopaedists), and physical and occupational therapists. Their goal is to treat all aspects of arthritis pain and help you learn to manage your pain. The physician, other health care professionals, and you, the patient, all play an active role in the management of arthritis pain.

How is Arthritis Pain Treated?

There is no single treatment that applies to all people with arthritis, but rather the doctor will develop a management plan designed to minimize your specific pain and improve the function of your joints. A number of treatments can provide short-term pain relief.

Short-Term Relief

- **Medications:** Because people with osteoarthritis have very little inflammation, pain relievers such as acetaminophen (Tylenol) may be effective. Patients with rheumatoid arthritis generally have pain caused by inflammation and often benefit from aspirin or other nonsteroidal antiinflammatory drugs (NSAIDs) such as ibuprofen.
- **Heat and cold:** The decision to use either heat or cold for arthritis pain depends on the type of arthritis and should be discussed with your doctor or physical therapist. Moist heat, such as a warm bath or shower, or dry heat, such as a heating pad, placed on the painful area of the joint for about 15 minutes may relieve the pain. An ice pack (or a

bag of frozen vegetables) wrapped in a towel and placed on the sore area for about 15 minutes may help to reduce swelling and stop the pain. If you have poor circulation, do not use cold packs.

- **Joint Protection:** Using a splint or a brace to allow joints to rest and protect them from injury can be helpful. Your physician or physical therapist can make recommendations.
- **Transcutaneous Electrical Nerve Stimulotion (TENS):** A small TENS device that directs mild electric pulses to nerve endings that lie beneath the skin in the painful area may relieve some arthritis pain. TENS seems to work by blocking pain messages to the brain and by modifying pain perception.
- **Massage:** In this pain-relief approach, a massage therapist will lightly stroke and/or knead the painful muscle. This may increase blood flow and bring warmth to a stressed area. However, arthritis-stressed joints are very sensitive so the therapist must be very familiar with the problems of the disease.
- **Acupuncture:** This procedure should only be done by a licensed acupuncture therapist. In acupuncture, thin needles are inserted at'specific points in the body. Scientists think that this stimulates the release of natural, pain-relieving chemicals produced by the brain or the nervous system.

Osteoarthritis and rheumatoid arthritis are chronic diseases that may last a lifetime. Learning how to manage your pain over the long term is an important factor in controlling the disease and maintaining a good quality of life. Following are some sources of long- term pain relief.

Long-Term Relief Medications

Nonsteroidal Anti-Inflammatory Drugs (NSAIDs): These are a class of drugs including aspirin and ibuprofen that are used to reduce pain and inflammation and may be used for both short-term and long-term relief in people with osteoarthritis and rheumatoid arthritis.

Disease-Modifying Anti-Rheumatic Drugs (DMARDS): These are drugs used to treat people with rheumatoid arthritis who have not responded to NSAIDs. Some of these include methotrexate, hydroxychloroquine-penicillamine and gold injections. These drugs are thought to influence and correct abnormalities of the immune system responsible for a disease like rheumatoid arthritis. Treatment with these medications requires careful monitoring by the physician to avoid side effects.

Corticosteroids: These are hormones that are very effective in treating arthritis. Corticosteroids can be taken by mouth or given by injection. Prednisone is the corticosteroid most often given by mouth to reduce the inflammation of rheumatoid arthritis. In both rheumatoid arthritis and osteoarthritis, the doctor also may inject a corticosteroid into the affected joint to stop pain. Because frequent injections may cause damage to the cartilage they should only be done once or twice a year.

- **Weight reduction:** Excess pounds put extra stress on weight-bearing joints such as the knees or hips. Studies have shown that overweight women who lost an average of 11 pounds substantially reduced the development of osteoarthritis in their knees. In addition, if osteoarthritis has already affected one knee, weight reduction will reduce the chance of it occurring in the other knee.
- **Exercise:** Swimming, walking, low-impact aerobic exercise and range-of- motion exercises may reduce joint pain and stiffness. In addition, stretching exercises are helpful. A physical therapist can help plan an exercise program that will give you the most benefit.
- **Surgery:** In select patients with arthritis, surgery may be necessary. The surgeon may perform an operation to

remove the synovium (synovectomy), realign the joint (osteotomy) or in advanced cases replace the damaged joint with an artificial one. Total joint replacement has provided not only dramatic relief from pain but also improvement in motion for many people with arthritis.

How can You Cope with Arthritis Pain?

The long-term goal of pain management is to help you cope with a chronic, often disabling disease. You may be caught in a cycle of pain, depression and stress. To break out of this cycle, you need to be an active participant with the doctor and other health care professionals in managing your pain. This may include physical therapy, cognitive-behavioural therapy, occupational therapy, biofeedback, relaxation techniques (for example, deep breathing and meditation), and family counselling therapy.

Another technique is to substitute distraction for pain. Focus your attention on things that you enjoy. Imagine a peaceful setting and wonderful physical sensations. Thinking about something that is enjoyable can help you relax and become less stressed. Find something that will make you laugh, a cartoon, a funny movie, or even a new joke. Try to put some joy back into your life. Even a small change in your mental image may break the pain cycle and provide relief.

What Research is being conducted on Arthritis Pain?

Recent NIAMS studies show that levels of several neuropeptides (compounds produced by cells of the nervous system), such as substance P, are increased in arthritic joints. Substance P is involved in the transmission of pain signals via the nervous system. At the University of Missouri, researchers are studying effects of substance P in the spines of animals with chronic arthritis. Findings from this study may be used to develop specific drugs for chronic pain such as that associated with arthritis.

Researchers are also studying the human knee and analyzing how injury in one joint may affect other joints. In addition, they are analysing the effect of pain and analgesics on gait (walking) and comparing pain and gait before and after surgical treatment of knee osteoarthritis.

• • •

9

Causes and Types of Knee Pain

Knee pain may subside on its own within a few days or persist for weeks or months. When the pain subsides within a few days, it is often due to minor problems such as a 'sprain'. When the knee pain persists for longer time, its causes can:

1. Pain due to injury to the knee;
2. Pain due to conditions not associated with injury.

Knee Sprain - causes and symptoms

- Common in day-to-day activities due to minor twisting or bending.
- Pain subsides within a few days to a week.
- Injury to semilunar cartilages.
- Caused when the knee is twisted or while landing on the knee suddenly.
- Pain may not subside within a few days.
- May give a feeling of something "getting stuck" or "loose" inside the knee.
- Knee may be locked in one position.

Injury to ligaments of the knee – causes and symptoms

- Front middle ligament often injured in sports when a sudden load comes on the knee or while jumping from a height.

- May also be due to forced twisting of the knee.
- May result in a 'sound' of something breaking inside the knee when the ligaments are injured.
- Rapid swelling of the knee because the blood fills the joint.

Fractures and Dislocations – Causes and Symptoms

Fractures may involve

- Lower end of the thigh bone
- Upper end of the bone or the kneecap
- Acute pain with immediate swelling
- Knee cap dislocation is common in adolescents
- Recurrent dislocation of knee cap is common

Overuse Injuries – Causes and Symptoms

- Common in sports persons and military recruits due to excessive demand on the joint.
- Pain occurs when adolescents or fresh military recruits undertake new or excessive physical activity.
- Injuries are usually due to a mild problem in the 'design' of the knee.
- Overuse injuries usually cause pain under stressful situation.

Injury to the knee is common in sports, accidents and sometimes day-to-day activities. It is a common cause of knee pain in younger people. There are several types or injuries to the knee joint such as tears in the meniscus, ligaments, etc. which are collectively known as 'Internal Derangement of the Knee' (or 'I.D.K.'). Sometimes it is difficult to diagnose the exact type of derangement, and therefore some people consider I.D.K. as synonymous with 'I Don't Know'.

Some causes of knee pain are not associated with injury and often cause pain in other joints also. The main group of diseases in this category is **arthritis.** The word "arthiritis" does not mean one disease – it means pain and swelling of a joint. There could be many reasons for this type of pain and swelling in the joint. It is important to remember that different types of arthritis occur at different ages and each one of them has a different outcome. Do not therefore worry unnecessarily if your doctor says that you have arthritis.

TYPES OF KNEE INJURY?

Injury to the knee joint is quite common. As mentioned earlier, this is because the design of the knee makes it relatively unstable. It is also prone to injuries because of the stress the knee is subjected to. Causes and symptoms of common knee injuries have been listed before. Described below are the management options for these injuries.

- **Knee Sprain:** Minor twisting or bending of the knee result in a sprain which indicates that some tissues around the knee are pulled. Since pain due to sprain subsides within a few days to a week, you should consult a doctor immediately if the pain persists for more than three weeks, or if the swelling around the knee increases steadily. Your doctor may recommend rest in a plaster cast or crepe bandage for a few weeks.
- **Injury to semilunar cartilages:** The inner half-moon shaped or semilunar cartilage is more likely to be injured than the outer cartilage. Although cartilage injuries may seem insignificant, they can cause considerable damage to the structures inside the knee. Your doctor may suspect a cartilage tear if the pain does not subside in a few days. If the knee gets 'locked' in one position consult a doctor immediately to free it by manual manipulation.

Most injuries to the knee can cause repeated complaints. It is often difficult to pinpoint the exact nature of the damage by knowing the history of the injury and examination of the knee joint. Your doctor may then suggest a procedure called "arthroscopy" in which the doctor looks directly into the joint through a thin pencil like tube called the arthroscope. The arthroscope is introduced into the knee through a small cut in the skin. A video-camera is attached to the arthroscope, which shows the inside of the knee on a television. Through this procedure, your doctor will be able to view all the corners of the joint and may therefore be able to identify the cause of symptoms and nature of damage. In most cases, the fault within the joint can be corrected by "key-hole-surgery" with the help of small instruments inserted through a few more small cuts. This often avoids a major operation, enables quick recovery and reduces hospital stay to less than forty eight hours. Arthroscopy not only helps in diagnosing a problem that was not diagnosed earlier but also provides a method of performing surgery with minimum cutting. This technique is therefore a boon for patients with joint problems. However, presently arthroscopy facility is available only at few centres in India.

- **Injury to ligaments of the knee:** Minor ligament tear such as sprain may heal on its own. If the tear in the ligament is complete or more than one ligament is torn at a time, the knee may not regain its normal strength. You may feel unstable from the day of the injury itself. If the front middle ligament alone is torn, there may not be any symptoms soon after the injury. After a period of time, you may feel 'weak' on the injured side and knee pain may develop. Most people with torn ligaments feel better with regular special exercises and careful movements of the knee in day to day activities. However, if the weakness persists, your doctor may recommend a major operation to replace the torn ligament with a new ligament constructed from other body tissues.

- **Fractures and dislocations:** X-rays of the knee are necessary to diagnose the extent of bone(s) damage due to the fracture. In most cases a major operation is necessary to fix the fractured pieces to their normal position with screws and steel plates. These steel plates result in normal movement at the knee. The pain and swelling subsides over a period of time.
- **Overuse injuries:** Knee injuries due to new or excessive physical activity is usually because of a mild problem in the 'design' of the knee. This problem may not routinely cause pain but can do so under stressful situations. It may not be necessary to give up physical activity that has resulted in knee pain. Instead, you should undertake strenuous physical activities only after receiving appropriate training and avoid excessive physical stress.

How is Arthritis of the knee Treated?

Most often osteoarthritis of the knee is treated with analgesics (pain-reducing medicines), such as aspirin or acetaminophen, NSAIds such as ibuprofen; and exercises to restore joint movement and strengthen the knee. Losing excess weight can also help people with osteoarthritis. Rheumatoid arthritis of the knee may require a treatment plan that includes physical therapy and use of more powerful medications. In people with arthritis of the knee, a seriously damaged joint may need to be surgically replaced with an artificial one.

• • •

10

Arthritis of the Shoulder

The shoulder joint is composed of three bones: the clavicle (collarbone), the scapula (shoulder blade), and the humerus (upper arm bone). Two joints facilitate shoulder movement. The acromioclavicular (AC) joint is located between the acromion (part of the scapula that forms the highest point of the shoulder) and the clavicle. The glenohumeral joint, commonly called the shoulder joint, is a ball-and-socket type joint that helps move the shoulder forward and backward and allows the arm to rotate in a circular fashion or hinge out and up away from the body. (The ball is the top, rounded portion of the upper arm bone or humerus; the socket or glenoid, is a dish-shaped part of the outer edge of the scapula into which the ball fits.) The capsule is a soft tissue envelope that encircles the glenohumeral joint. It is lined by a thin, smooth synovial membrane.

The bones of the shoulder are held in place by muscles, tendons, and ligaments. Tendons are tough cords of tissue that attach the shoulder muscles to bone and assist the muscles in moving the shoulder. Ligaments attach shoulder bones to each other, providing stability. For example, the front of the joint capsule is anchored by three glenohumeral ligaments.

The rotator cuff is a structure composed of tendons that with associated muscles, holds the ball at the top of the humerus in the glenoid socket and provides mobility and strength to the shoulder joint. Two sac-like structures called bursae permit smooth gliding between bone, muscle and tendon. They cushion and protect the rotator cuff from the bony arch of the acromion.

What are the Origin and Causes of Shoulder Problems?

The shoulder is the most movable joint in the body. However, it is an unstable joint because of the range of motion allowed. It is easily subject to injury because the ball of the upper arm is larger than the shoulder socket that holds it. To remain stable, the shoulder must be anchored by its muscles, tendons and ligaments. Some shoulder problems arise from the disruption of these soft tissues as a result of injury or from: overuse or underuse of the shoulder. Other problems arise from a degenerative process in which tissues break down and no longer function well.

Shoulder pain may be localized or may be referred to areas around the shoulder or down the arm. Disease within the body (such as gallbladder, liver, or heart disease, or disease of the cervical spine of the neck) also may generate pain that travels along nerves to the shoulder.

What is Arthritis of the Shoulder?

Arthritis is a degenerative disease caused by either wear and tear (osteoarthritis) or an inflammation (rheumatoid arthritis) of one or more joints. Arthritis not only affects joints; it may secondarily affect supporting structures such as muscles, tendons and ligaments.

What are the Signs of Shoulder Arthritis and how is it Diagnosed?

The usual signs of arthritis of the shoulder are pain, particularly over the AC joint, and a decrease in shoulder motion.

A doctor may suspect the patient has arthritis when there is both pain and swelling in the joint. The diagnosis may be confirmed by a physical examination and x-rays. Blood tests may be helpful for diagnosing rheumatoid arthritis, but other tests may be needed as well. Analysis of synovial fluid from the shoulder joint may be helpful in diagnosing some kinds of arthritis. Although arthroscopy permits direct visualization of damage to cartilage, tendons and ligaments, and may confirm a diagnosis, it is usually only done if a repair procedure is to be performed.

How is Pain (Arthritis) of the Shoulder Treated?

Most often osteoarthritis of the shoulder is treated with nonsteroidal anti- inflammatory drugs Such as aspirin or ibuprofen. (Rheumatoid arthritis of the shoulder may require physical therapy and additional medicine, such as corticosteroids.) When conservative treatment of osteoarthritis of the shoulder fails to relieve pain or improve function, or when there is severe deterioration of the joint causing parts to loosen and move out of place, shoulder joint replacement (arthroplasty) may provide better results. In this operation, a surgeon replaces the shoulder joint with an artificial ball for the humerus and a cap (glenoid) for the scapula. Passive shoulder exercises (where someone else moves the arm to rotate the shoulder joint) are started soon after surgery. Patients begin exercising on their own about 3 to 6 weeks after surgery. Eventually, stretching and strengthening exercises become a major part of the rehabilitation program. The success of the operation often depends on the condition of rotator cuff muscles prior to surgery and the degree to which the patient follows the exercise program.

• • •

11

Rheumatoid Arthritis

Rheumatoid arthritis is a disease in which the body develops 'allergy' to some components of the blood. These components accumulate in the joints and some other parts of the body. The body's natural defence mechanism reacts adversely to this accumulation. The result is swelling and pain. Rheumatoid arthritis can cripple a person rapidly, is often extensive and may sometimes even be life-threatening. It is more common in women twenty to forty years of age and may run in families.

Symptoms

Early symptoms of rheumatoid arthritis are fever with vague aches and pains in the body including the joints. After about four to six weeks the symptoms are more severe and the pain is present in several joints, especially the joints of the hands and feet. Knee is a major joint and is therefore usually affected. Walking may become difficult. If you do not walk enough, your thigh muscles may become wasted or thin. Rheumatoid arthritis may affect various systems of the body such as the eyes, lungs and the heart. Severity of the symptoms of rheumatoid arthritis is not constant. The symptoms may completely disappear and appear again after some time.

You should consult with a doctor as soon as possible if you have pain and swelling one or more joints. It is important to remember that all joint pains and swelling are not due to rheumatoid arthritis.

What is the Difference Between Osteoarthritis and Rheumatoid Arthritis?

Osteoarthritis usually begins after the age of forty years over a period of several years. It usually begins on joints on one side of the body. It usually affects joints in the knee, hips, hands, feet and the backbone. There are no associated symptoms such as fatigue, fever or loss of weight.

Rheumatoid arthritis starts between twenty five to forty years of age and the symptoms may appear and disappear without any warning. It affects joints on both sides of the body at the same time. It affects most joints including knuckles, wrist and elbows. Rheumatoid arthritis is usually accompanied with fever, weight loss and fatigue.

Laboratory Tests

Your doctor may recommend a test called the R.A. factor. Although this test often helps in diagnosis, it is not always reliable. This is because it is occasionally positive in people who do not have rheumatoid arthritis. Your doctor will therefore diagnose your condition on the basis of history; physical examination and laboratory tests.

Management

The basic principles for management of rheumatoid arthritis and other associated diseases. These include:

- **Correct Diagnosis:** Since rheumatoid arthritis is just one type of arthritis which involves multiple joints, it is important for you to consult with a doctor, especially a joint-disease specialist (Rheumatologist) and trust his/her judgment. Your doctor may not be able to make the diagnosis before six weeks.

- **Patient education:** Since rheumatoid arthritis is potentially crippling, it is important for you to avoid anxiety. Your doctor will give you details about the course of the disease such as its fluctuating course, long-term treatment options, need to use more than one medicines which may have several adverse impacts, cost of treatment and the need to consult the doctor regularly. You can limit the adverse impacts of the disease by following your doctors recommendations.
- **Avoid treatment from doctors who are not qualified:** Several selfstyled doctors may promise your magic cure for rheumatoid arthritis. It is however important to remember that although some medicines may be partially effective for other types of arthritis, rheumatoid arthritis requires a well-planned management schedule.
- **Avoid steroids:** Steroids are chemical substances produced by some glands in the body. They are also available as medicines. Although steroids may give immediate relief you will require larger and larger dose to relieve symptoms over a period of time. They have serious side-effects on almost all parts of the body. Of these, weight-gain, swelling of the face, excess hair growth on the face, reduced vision due to cataract, ulcers and weakness of bones are more common.
- **Diet:** Rheumatoid arthritis does not require any special diet. Avoiding some food items are not likely to cure the disease. You may however have loss of appetite and anaemia. You should therefore eat a balanced diet preferably as small and frequent meals.
- **Moderate activity:** Bed rest is not necessary, except in early painful stages of the disease. Once this phase is over, you should start normal joint movements.

- **Physiotherapy:** It is very important to start physiotherapy after the disease is controlled a little by medicines. Physiotherapy helps to regain joint mobility and strength. You can do the recommended exercise and heat therapy yourself after learning the correct technique from a qualified person.

Principles of Management

Correct diagnosis, preferably by a rheumatologist.

Education regarding the course of illness and adverse effects of the disease and its management options.

Acceptance that the disease is not curable.

Avoid steroids.

Eat small frequent balanced meals.

Do simple exercise after the painful stage subsides and gradually increase its duration.

Learn the correct technique of physiotherapy including exercise from a trained professional.

Avoid exercise from which you cannot recover within one hour.

Normal sexual activity can be practiced, especially when the painful stage subsides.

Avoid pregnancy during active phase of the disease.

Consult your doctor regularly for modifications in your treatment schedule depending upon your condition.

Surgery such as knee replacement if all other methods for joint mobility have failed.

Exercise

Exercise help to relieve and prevent joint stiffness, muscle weakness, joint deformity and dependence on others. You should however avoid excessive bending of the joints. Increase the intensity and duration of the exercise gradually as you may feel tired after doing exercises to regain joint mobility and muscle strength. A simple rule is that you should recover from the 'strain' within one hour of exercises. It is important to find a correct balance between rest and exercise.

Three types of exercises help:

- those which maintain or increase joint mobility;
- those which improve muscle strength; and
- those which increase the general health and are beneficial to the heart and the lungs.
- **Marriage, sexual activity and motherhood:** Rheumatoid arthritis is a chronic disease which limits your ability to do normal work over a period of years. You can be sexual active although it may be difficult when you have joint pains. Although pregnancy is not contra-indicated in rheumatoid arthritis it is better to avoid pregnancy during the active phase of the disease when you require long-term medicines. Rarely the hip joint may be affected and therefore sexual activity and delivery may be difficult.
- **Regulate treatment schedule under doctor's guidance:** There is no common treatment for rheumatoid arthritis. Your doctor is likely to recommend a combination of medicines depending upon the severity of your disease, your body's acceptance of the medicines and their side-effects. Your doctor may have to modify the treatment schedule frequently in the initial stages till the correct combination and dose is achieved.
- **Surgery**: Your doctor may recommend surgery after other methods of preserving the joint and making it usable have failed. Knee joint replacement has become a very standard operation as it makes you mobile even after a prolonged illness.

MODERATE TREATMENT

When we use the term moderate it implies that it is a scaled down version of a radical treatment so far discussed.

Morning keep the bowel clean with the help of a non violent enema.

Herbal paste/juice can be combined with the vegetable juice of banana stem and/or ash pumpkin.

If time permits spinal bath combined with hot foot bath may be taken for 15-20 minutes. Full bath in bearable cold water is to be followed.

With the above oral medicine the patient may proceed to his/her place of work/studies or continue with his/her light household chores.

10-11 a.m. Depending upon the convenience in the place of work/studies the patient may take some tender coconut water or some fresh non citrus fruits or some vegetable juice. If none of the above are available; plain cold water is sufficient.

Lunch at home: Some fresh vegetables and some conservatively cooked vegetables, with the usual garnishings of coconut scrapings, coriander leaves etc. may be taken. Better to avoid cereals.

If going to work some fruits or fresh vegetables are prescribed. Cooked food would have become very stale. Further he/she is expected to continue the work, also in the afternoon.

If at home a spinal bath with hot water foot bath may be taken in the afternoon. Those who go out for work/studies are advised to take a spinal bath with/without hot water foot bath without fail on return. Whatever help is needed for getting into the tub and getting up should be obtained. A glass of tender coconut water is an ideal drink in the evening.

Night dinner may consist of some unrefined cereals and conservatively cooked vegetables.

Before retiring to bed he/she may apply some edible herbal oil on the affected joints. This will be followed with an alternate hot and cold fomentation and at the end of it apply a stimulating wet pack on the affected joint(s).

• • •

12

Juvenile Rheumatoid Arthritis

Juvenile rheumatoid arthritis (JRA) is a different form of arthritis that causes joint inflammation and stiffness for more than 6 weeks in a child of 16 years of age or less. Inflammation causes redness, swelling, warmth, and soreness in the joints, although many children with JRA do not complain of joint pain. Any joint can be affected and inflammation may limit the mobility of affected joints. Doctors classify three kinds of JRA by the number of joints involved, the symptoms, and the presence or absence of certain antibodies in the blood. (Antibodies are special proteins made by the immune system.) These classifications help the doctor determine how the disease will progress.

Pauciarticular: (paw-see-are-tick- you-Iar): Pauciarticular means that four or fewer joints are affected. Pauciarticular is the most common form of JRA; about half of all children with JRA have this type. Pauciarticular disease typically affects large joints, such as the knees. Girls under the age of 15 yrs. are most likely to develop this type of JRA.

Some children have special proteins in the blood called antinuclear antibodies (ANAs). Eye disease affects about 20 to 30 percent of children with pauciarticular JRA. Up to 80 percent of those with eye disease also test positive for ANA and the disease tends to develop at a particularly early age in these children. Regular examinations by an ophthalmologist (a doctor who specializes in eye diseases) are necessary to prevent serious eye problems such as iritis (inflammation of the iris) or uveitis (inflammation of the inner eye or uvea). Many children with pauciarticular disease outgrow arthritis by adulthood, although eye problems can continue and joint symptoms may recur in some people.

Polyarticular: About 30 percent of all children with JRA have polyarticular disease. In polyarticular disease, five or more joints are affected. The small joints, such as those in the hands and feet, are most commonly involved, but the disease may also affect large joints. Polyarticular JRA often is symmetrical, that is, it affects the same joint on both sides of the body. Some children with polyarticular disease have a special kind of antibody in their blood called IgM rheumatoid factor (RF). These children often have a more severe form of the disease, which doctors consider to be the same as adult rheumatoid arthritis.

Systemic: Besides joint swelling, the systemic form of JRA is characterized by fever and a light pink rash, and may also affect internal organs such as the heart, liver, spleen and lymph nodes. Doctors sometimes call it Still's disease. Almost all children with this type of JRA test negative for both RF and ANA. The systemic form affects 20 percent of all children with JRA. A small percentage of these children develop arthritis in many joints and can have severe arthritis that continues into adulthood.

JRA is an autoimmune disorder, which means that the body mistakenly identifies some of its own cells and tissues as foreign. The immune system, which normally helps to fight off harmful, foreign substances such as bacteria or viruses, begins to attack healthy cells and tissues. The result is inflammation-marked by redness, heat, pain and swelling. Doctors do not know why the immune system goes awary in children who develop JRA.

Scientists suspect that it is a two-step process. First something in a child's genetic makeup gives them a tendency to develop JRA; and then an environmental factor, such as a virus, triggers the development of JRA.

The most common symptom of all types of JRA is persistent joint swelling, pain, and stiffness that typically is worse in the morning or after a nap. The pain may limit movement of the affected joint although many children, especially younger ones, will not complain of pain. JRA commonly affects the knees and joints in the hands and feet. One of the earliest signs of JRA may be limping in the morning because of an affected knee. Besides joint symptoms, children with systemic JRA have a high fever and a light pink rash. The rash and fever may appear and disappear very quickly. Systemic JRA also may cause the lymph nodes located in the neck and other parts of the body to swell. In some cases (less than half), internal organs including the heart and very rarely, the lungs may be involved. Eye inflammation is a potentially severe complication that sometimes occurs in children with pauciarticular IRA. Eye diseases such as iritis and uveitis often are not present until some time after a child first develops JRA. Typically, there are periods when the symptoms of JRA are better or disappear (remissions) and times when symptoms are worse (flares). JRA is different in each child-some may have just one or two flares and never have symptoms again, while others experience many flares or even have symptoms that never go away.

The Difference between JRA and Adult RA: The main difference between juvenile and adult rheumatoid arthritis is that many people with JRA outgrow the illness, while adults usually have lifelong symptoms. Studies estimate that by adulthood, JRA symptoms disappear in more than half of all affected children. Additionally, unlike rheumatoid arthritis in an adult, JRA may affect bone development as well as the child's growth. Another difference between JRA and adult rheumatoid arthritis is the percentage of people who are positive for RF. About 70 to 80 percent of all adults with rheumatoid arthritis are positive for RF, but fewer than half of all children with rheumatoid arthritis are RF positive. Presence of RF indicates an increased chance that Juvenile Rheumatoid Arthritis will continue into adulthood.

• • •

13

Exercise for Arthritics / Pain

Many arthritics shirk from exercise because they think it would be terribly painful in their condition. But in arthritis, if moving hurts, not moving destroys. Incorrect moving harms but intelligent moving heals. Use it or lose it!

Exercise helps keep you fit and slim. If you have arthritis, it helps keep your joints, muscles and bones healthy. Exercise also gives you more energy to keep up with daily activities. However, the pain and swelling of arthritis may complicate your workout routine, and hence the need for a trained physical therapist. A yoga teacher can train you in movements with proper joint alignment which help bring deformed joints back to normal position as appropriate muscles are lengthened and strengthened.

The amount and form of exercise recommended for each individual will vary depending on which joints are involved, the amount of inflammation, how stable the joints are, and whether a joint replacement procedure has been done. A skilled physician who is knowledgeable about the medical and rehabilitation needs of people with arthritis, working with a physical therapist also familiar with the needs of people with arthritis, can design an exercise plan for each patient.

Should People with Arthritis Exercise?

Yes. Studies have shown that exercise helps people with arthritis in many ways. Exercise reduces joint pain and stiffness and increases flexibility, muscle strength, and endurance. It also helps with weight reduction and contributes to an improved sense of well-being.

How does Exercise Fit into a Treatment Plan for People with Arthritis?

Exercise is one part of a comprehensive arthritis treatment plan. Treatment plans also may include rest and relaxation, proper diet, medication, and instruction about proper use of joints and ways to conserve energy (that is, not waste motion) as well as the use of pain relief methods.

How does a Person with Arthritis Start an Exercise Program?

People with arthritis should discuss exercise options with their doctors. Most doctors recommend exercise for their patients. Many people with arthritis begin with easy, range-of-motion exercises and low-impact aerobics. People with arthritis can participate in a variety of, but not all, sports and exercise programs. The doctor will know which, if any, sports are off limits.

The doctor may have suggestions about how to get started or may refer the patient to a physical therapist. It is best to find a physical therapist who has experience working with people who have arthritis. The therapist will design an appropriate home exercise program and teach clients about pain-relief methods, proper body mechanics (placement of the body for a given task, such as lifting a heavy box), joint protection, and conserving energy.

What Types of Exercise are most Suitable for Someone with Arthritis?

- Isometric Exercises consist of tightening your muscles without moving your joints. Example: From an upright sitting or standing position, press the palms of both hands together with all your might, as if you were trying to press communion wafers. This strengthens your arm muscles.
- Isotonic Exercises strengthen muscles by using a light weight or other resistance. Several studies now show that if you improve muscle strength, you decrease pain. An example of isotonic exercises for your thighs: Sit in a chair high enough that you can swing your leg. Keep your thigh on the chair and straighten out your knee. Hold a few seconds. Then bend your knee back as far as possible. Repeat with the other knee.
- Range of Motion Exercises reduce stiffness and help keep your joints flexible by making sure they are regularly moved the full extent of their range. Example for your thumbs: Open your hand with your fingers straight. Reach your thumb across your palm until it touches the base of the little finger. Then stretch your thumb out and repeat.

Keep in mind that normal every day activities, such as cleaning, climbing stairs, dressing, bathing, cooking, lifting, or bending do not move your joints through their entire range of motion. If your joints are very painful and swollen, do not forgo your exercises. Simply move them gently through their range of motion.

- Aerobic exercises improve cardiovascular fitness, help control weight, and improve overall function. Weight control can be important to people who have arthritis because extra weight puts extra pressure on many joints. Some studies show that aerobic exercise can reduce inflammation in some joints.

How to Get Started

- Discuss exercise plans with your doctor.
- Start with supervision from a physical therapist.
- Apply heat to sore joints (optional; many people with arthritis start their exercise program this way).
- Stretch and warm up with range-of-motion exercises.
- Start strengthening exercises slowly with small weights (a kilo weight can make a big difference).
- Progress slowly.
- Use cold packs after exercising (optional; many people with arthritis complete their exercise routine this way).
- Add aerobic exercise.
- Consider appropriate recreational exercise (after doing range of-motion, strengthening, and aerobic exercise). Fewer injuries to arthritic joints occur during recreational exercise if it is preceded by strengthening and aerobic exercise that gets your body in the best condition possible.
- Ease off if joints become painful, inflamed, or red and work with your doctor to find the cause and eliminate it.
- Choose the exercise program you enjoy most and make it a habit.
- Avoid weight bearing activities such as climbing stairs and prolonged walking

Pain Relief Methods?

There are known methods to stop pain for short periods of time. This temporary relief can make it easier for people who have arthritis to exercise. The following methods have worked for many people:

- Moist heat supplied by warm towels, hot packs, a bath, or a shower can be used at home for 15 to 20 minutes three times a day to relieve symptoms. A health professional can use short waves, microwaves, and ultrasound to deliver deep heat to non inflamed joint areas. Deep heat is not recommended for patients with acutely inflamed joints. Deep heat is often used around the shoulder to relax tight tendons prior to stretching exercises.

- Cold supplied by a bag of ice or frozen vegetables wrapped in a towel helps to stop pain and reduce swelling when used.
- 10 to 15 minutes at a time, it is often used for acutely inflamed joints. People who have Raynauds phenomenon should not use this method.
- Application of a muscle ointment at night before going to bed helps people with arthritis to feel much better all day. They aren't stiff when they wake up in the morning
- Massages, on account of the gentle warmth they produce, alleviate the pain considerably. In case of stiff joints, massage with a mixture of warm coconut and mustard oil and camphor.

Work the muscles that are attached to the tendons leading to your painful joints. For example if you have arthritis in your hands then work the forearms from the wrists to the elbows, using a compression technique. To do this use with the heel of your hand, your thumb or your elbow to press down on the muscle and hold it for several seconds, then release. For arthritis of the foot, work the calf and the front to the leg.

- Mobilisation therapies include traction (gentle, steady pulling), massage, and manipulation (using the hands to restore normal movement to stiff joints). When done by a trained professional, these methods can help control pain and increase joint motion and muscle and tendon flexibility.

- TENS (transcutaneous electrical nerve stimulation) and biofeedback are two additional methods that may provide some pain relief, but many patients find that they cost too much money and take too much time.
- Relaxation therapy also helps reduce pain. Patients can learn to release the tension in their muscles to relieve pain. Physical therapists may be able to teach relaxation techniques.
- Acupuncture is a traditional Chinese method of pain relief. A medically qualified acupuncturist places needles in certain sites. Researchers believe that the needles stimulate deep sensory nerves that tell the brain to release natural painkillers (endorphins). Acupressure is similar to acupuncture, but pressure is applied to the acupuncture sites instead of using needles.

How Often Should People with Arthritis Exercise?

- Range-of-motion exercises can be done daily and should be done at least every other day.
- Strengthening exercises can also be done daily and should be done at least every other day unless you have severe pain or swelling in your joints.
- Endurance exercises should be done for 20 to 30 minutes three times a week unless you have severe pain or swelling in your joints.

What Type of Strengthening Program is Best?

This varies depending on personal preference, the type of arthritis involved, and how active the inflammation is. Strengthening one's muscles can help take the burden off painful joints. Strength training can be done with small weights, exercise machines, isometrics, elastic bands, and resistive water exercises: Correct positioning is critical, because if done incorrectly, strengthening exercises can cause muscle tears, more pain, and more joint swelling.

Are there Different Exercises for People with Different Types of Arthritis?

There are many types of arthritis. Experienced doctors, physical therapists and occupational therapists can recommend exercises that are particularly helpful for a specific type of arthritis. Doctors and therapists also know specific exercises for particularly painful joints. There may be exercises that are offlimits for people with a particular type of arthritis or when joints are swollen and inflamed. People with arthritis should discuss their exercise plans with a doctor. Doctors who treat people with arthritis include rheumatologists, general practitioners, family doctors, internists, and rehabilitation specialists.

How Much Exercise is too Much?

Most experts agree that if exercise causes pain that lasts for more than 1 hour, it is too much. People with arthritis should work with their physical therapist or doctor to adjust their exercise program when they notice any of the following signs of too much exercise:

- Unusual or persistent fatigue
- Increased weakness
- Decreased range of motion
- Increased joint swelling
- Continuing pain (pain that lasts more than 1 hour after exercising)

Exercises to Keep Your Muscles from Becoming Stiff

If you have trouble sitting for long periods of time, try the following exercises devised by physiologist Mary Sampey. These are useful for keeping your muscles from becoming stiff. Always begin these exercises by sitting comfortably, but alertly in your chair, feet flat on the floor and hands resting on your thighs. Each exercise should be done as tolerated, however only a few minutes at a time are necessary to make a difference.

Neck Stretch: Gently bend your head forward, then to each side. Repeat 2 to 3 times.

Arm Reaches: Sitting up straight, stretch your arms over your head. Reach first with your right arm, then with your left, as if you were climbing a ladder. If you can repeat this set of stretches 9 to 10 times.

Wrist Rolls: Gently rotate your right wrist. Circle in one direction several times, then reverse the rotation. Repeat with your left wrist.

Shoulder Rolls: Sitting up straight, slowly roll your shoulders in a circle. Roll forward 2 to 3 times, then backward.

Side Circles: Stretch arms out to your sides. Circle forward 10 times, starting with small, tight circles that gradually become broader and looser. Repeat with reverse circling.

Lower Back Stretch: Slowly bend your upper body toward your knees as low as comfortably possible, letting your arms rest on your lower legs or around your ankles. Return to the sitting position, then repeat 1 to 2 times.

Upper Body Stretch: Visualize a wire attached to the top of your head, gently stretching your body upward. Hold the stretch for a few moments, then relax. Repeat 2 to 3 times.

Tiptoe Stretches: Sit with your feet flat on the floor. Leaving the front part of the foot (ball and toes) on the floor, slowly raise the heel of your right foot into a comfortable stretch. You should feel a slight stretch in your calf as well. Then lower your heel back to the floor. Repeat 2 to 3 times with your right foot.

Heel Stretches: Sit with feet flat on the floor. Leaving the heel of your foot on the floor, slowly raise the front part of your foot a few inches until you feel gently stretch in your ankle and calf. Then lower the front part of your foot back to the floor. Repeat 2 to 3 times, then switch to the left foot.

• • •

14

Diet and Nutritional Supplements

If you thought that all you could do to combat arthritis was to pop painkillers and suffer, you obviously have not been talking to the right people. There are enough good studies to show that diet therapy may improve symptoms in some cases.

- Corn, wheat, cow's milk, pork, oranges, oats, eggs, beef, coffee, cheese, grapefruit, lemon, tomato, groundnuts and soya are the foods most likely to cause arthritis. Makes sense to avoid them, doesn't it?

Note: Animal products such as meat and cows' dairy products contain a fatty acid called Arachidonic acid that greatly contributes to the inflammation of joints).

- Diet should be planned on alkaline lines so as to rid the system of its toxicity. A diet predominated by raw salad, sprouts and cooked vegetables is effective in this regard. At least one meal a day should be exclusively comprised of raw salad, sprouts and fruits. Excess salt should be avoided as salt will cause more water to be retained in the body and joint pains will increase.
- A weekly fast for a day or two, or at least a juice fast for a couple of days, is extremely beneficial. Constipation should be avoided since any increase in toxicity only irritates the joints and causes further inflammation.

- Make it a point to include cabbage, carrot, cucumber, lettuce, onion, radish, beetroot, cauliflower, banana, and green leafy vegetables in your salad or in your vegetable menu. Eat enough garlic as it is very effective in removing toxins and stimulating blood circulation. Above all, avoid all refined foods, flesh foods, eggs, milk and milk products and fried and spicy foods.
- Tomatoes, white potatoes, eggplant and green bell peppers are members of the Night Shade Vegetable Family. These vegetables contain a chemical called Soltanine that may aggravate arthritis sufferers. Elimination of these vegetables for one week and the reintroduction of one - of these at a time, may determine any possible allergic reaction.
- Omega-3 polyunsaturated fatty acids (PUFAs) could help prevent and treat a wide range of diseases, including arthritis. The daily requirement is probably around a teaspoon of essential fatty acids a day. Fish is a rich source of omega-3 PUF and also of eicosapentaenoic acid (EPA). EPA greatly reduces inflammation and contributing allergic responses. If you are a vegetarian, use Flax Seed Oil (Omega 3 oi1) or canola oil (high in a plant form of omega-3 alpha linoleic fatty acid).
- Take in plenty of berries (cherries, blueberries). These are rich in flavonoids that inhibit histaminic release and reduces the inflammatory response.
- Take enough of vitamin C daily. This vitamin assists in decreasing histaminic levels and inflammation while providing anti-oxidant effects. Vitamin C is a marker for fruits and vegetables rich in other healing compounds. Therefore, stick with foods high in vitamin C rather than supplements. Indian gooseberry (aamla) is one of the best known sources of vitamin C.

- **Enzymes:** Especially Trypsin, Bromelain and Quercetin along with Vitamin C and Flavanoids, have been found to provide a wider use for individuals with Rheumatoid Arthritis than non-steroidal drugs such as aspirin.
- **Acidophillus:** Provides friendly bacteria to balance abnormal intestinal flora common with Rheumatoid Arthritis sufferers.
- Because RA follows a pattern of flare ups, it's natural to suspect you are allergic to what you have just eaten. Keep a daily chart of your diet and your reactions; this will help you eliminate the food type to which you are allergic.

Fat Intake & Arthritis

According to Prevention, the immune substances that inflame your joints are made from the kind of fat you eat. Linoleic acid - the predominant polyunsaturated fat in most vegetable oils such as soyabean, corn oil, safflower and sunflower, generate some of the most inflammatory immune substances. Therefore change your fatty-acid profile to a less inflammatory one. Canola oil is once again preferable. It will also help keep your cholesterol profile in check.

A low-fat diet (keep fat at 20 percent of total calories) has been found to decrease morning stiffness by 50 percent and improve walking time by 30 percent.

Suggested Calcium & Vitamin D Intake

On the basis of the most current information available, optimal calcium intake is estimated to be 400 mg/day (birth to 6 months) to 600 mg/day (6 to 12 months) in infants; 800 mg/day in young children (1 to 5 years) and 800 to 1,200 mg/day for older children (6 to 10 years); 1,200 to 1,500 mg/day for adolescents and young adults (11 to 24 years); 1,000 mg/day for women between 25 and 50 years; 1,200 to 1,500 mg/day for pregnant or lactating women; and 1,000 mg/day for postmenopausal women on estrogen replacement therapy and 1,500 mg/day for postmenopausal women not on estrogen therapy. Recommended daily intake for men is 1,000 mg/day (25 to 65 years). For all women and men over 65, daily intake is recommended to be 1,500 mg/day, although further research is needed in this age group. These guidelines are based upon calcium from the diet plus any calcium taken in supplemental form.

Also remember that adequate vitamin D is essential for optimal calcium absorption. More so in osteoarthritis which breaks down cartilage in a joint, causing the underlying bone to be subjected to greater stress. Low levels of vitamin D may impair the ability of bone to respond to this increased wear and tear. Take multivitamin with at least 4000 IU of vitamin D.

- Phosphorus is an element which takes out excess of calcium from body. So, make sure its proper bone should be consumed.
- If there is RA or any related disorder, diet should be suggested by a qualified nutritional therapist.

• • •

15

What is Osteoarthritis?

Osteoarthritis is destruction of the smooth cartilage covering the ends of the bones. This destruction is similar to the wear and tear of moving machines. It usually starts in the middle age without any specific cause. You may have seen elderly persons walking like a duck, or using a stick to walk. Most of these people suffer from osteoarthritis.

Stages

In early stages there is pain or catch in the knee while:

- getting up from sitting position; or
- changing position of the knee after a period of rest in one position;
- in later stages, pain is almost constant and becomes worse on exertion. At this stage the pain is relieved by :
- rest;
- pain killer medicines; or
- oil massage.

In advanced stage, walking is difficult and often needs a lot of effort. Going up and down the stairs is especially very difficult. The knee may appear 'swollen' and thigh may appear thin. The shape of the legs changes and the knee bows outwards. At this stage, the gait changes and there may be sideways lurch at every step.

Causes

Common causes of osteoarthritis are:

- Wear-and-tear due to prolonged use of the joint (This is the commonest cause of osteoarthritis);
- Defect in quality of the cartilage such as in a disease called pseudogout;
- Defect in alignment of the articulating surfaces;
- Loose structures inside the joint such as a loose cover of the meniscus;
- Old injury; and
- Previous infection.

Risk groups

Osteoarthritis may run in families. It is more common in obese people and those who use the knee excessively such as for sports, standing for a long time or working for long hours with knee in extreme positions. Osteoarthritis is 10 times more common in females than in the males. People with bowed legs develop osteoarthritis much earlier.

Symptoms

Osteoarthritis of the knee is more common among people above fifty years of age, especially the obese. Most people with osteoarthritis complain of pain and/or creaking sound in the knee.

Many people who believe that knee pain means beginning of old age do not always consult with a doctor. It is important to remember that knee pain can occur at all ages and some causes are curable. Also, there are some diseases which may start as a mild pain but rapidly progress to destroy the knee joint. Early diagnosis and timely management that can prevent the progress of an otherwise progressive disease.

When to consult with a Doctor?

You should consult with a doctor, especially orthopaedic surgeon if you have:

- Pain or stiffness in one joint only or if one joint is affected more than the other;
- Repeated swelling of the knee with pain;
- Symptoms suggestive of a mechanical fault as sudden clicking, something either moving or loose inside the joint.
- Recent bowing of the legs with pain or the inner side of the knee.
- Walking about within the house is difficult due to pain.

Management

Osteoarthritis is not curable. Once it starts, it remains for rest of the life. However, you can relieve the symptoms and minimise disability with timely treatment. Management of osteoarthritis is through

- non-surgical methods in early stages and
- surgical methods in advanced stages.

Non-Surgical Management

The patient has to do the following for non-surgical management of osteoarth ritis.

Patient education: You may start worrying about being crippled because of arthritis. Your doctor will, therefore, give you a very true picture of your condition which will help lessen your fears and anxiety.

Weight reduction: Regular and adequate exercise may be a problem if you have difficulty in walking. You may, however, do cycling or swimming regularly. It is, therefore, important to modify your diet and avoid high calorie foods such as sugar, sweets, rice, potato, oil or ghee.

Avoid the following which put excessive Stress on the Knee

- Sitting on the floor, in low chairs, sofa or beds.
- Squatting, sitting cross-legged and using Indian style toilets.
- Exercises in which you have stand or walk for a long time.

You may get Relief by

- Doing exercises where you can sit on a chair or stool.
- Doing specific exercises to build up the muscles around the knee for providing support to the 'weak' knee.
- Occasional use of medicines to relieve pain. Paracetamol is a safer medicine.

Surgical Management

Three types of surgeries are recommended for management of osteoarthritis. These include:

- arthroscopy;
- Correction of the alignment of the knee; and
- changing the knee joint. None of these surgeries cure osteoarthritis. Your doctor may recommend anyone of these options depending upon the condition of your knee.
- **Arthroscopy:** Your doctor may recommend if you either have
- mechanical problems such as something stuck or loose inside the joint or
- repeated swelling of the knee joint. Although the relief may be partial or temporary, it is often recommended because it is a safe and 'minor' procedure.

As mentioned earlier, your doctor can view the inside of the knee directly through an arthroscope and assess the condition of the cartilage covering the bone-ends and the semi-lunar cartilages. Your doctor will also be able to remove (a) any loose or torn pieces of semi-lunar or articular cartilages or

- loose or over-grown tissue lining the knee. The joint will then be washed thoroughly with saline water to completely remove damaged pieces.
- **Correction of alignment of the knee.** Your doctor may suggest a surgery called High Tibial Osteotomy (HTO) to correct the alignment of the knee. This surgery is usually recommended if you have painful osteoarthritis of the knee with bowing of the legs. When your legs are bowed, more body weight passes through the inner side than the outer side of the knee. During the surgery the bone just below the knee is cut and realigned so that the more body weight passes through the outer side of the knee. After this surgery more than seventy percent patients have relief from pain for almost eight to ten years. It is effective for mild to moderate arthritis, and people who are either young or not obese.

High tibial osteotomy or HTO is a major surgery and requires a plaster cast for a month after the operation. You can however start walking to the toilet with the plaster about one week after the surgery. Your doctor will also recommend physiotherapy for a few weeks after the cast is removed.

- **Changing the knee joint:** This is a relatively new technique in which the damaged ends of the bones of the knee joint are removed and replaced with artificial parts. A cup-like part is fixed on the end of the thigh bone and a plate-like part is fixed on the end of the leg bone with a special glue called bone-cement. The new parts of the knee are smooth and therefore there is no pain during normal movements of the joint. Although this surgery gives instant relief from pain, it is not always effective. You may have to observe several restrictions in movements so that the new joint may last for five to eight years. Also, the artificial knee joint is very expensive. This surgery is usually recommended for people who are not able to walk within the house also.

• • •

16

Other Conditions Like Arthritis

These are same disorders which resemble to arthritis.

Bursitis and Tendinitis

Bursitis and Tendinitis result from irritation caused by injuring or overusing a joint. Bursitis affects a small sac that helps muscles more easily. Tendinitis affects the tendons that attach muscle to bone.

Polymyalgia Rheumatica (PMR)

This rheumatic disorder causes muscle pain, aching and stiffness in the neck and shoulders, lower back, thighs and hips. It can last a few months or many years. Most people experience severe stiffness in the morning.

Fibromyalgia

People with fibromyalgia feel pain and stiffness in muscles and tendons, especially in the neck and upper back. The pain can last for weeks, months or years. The symptoms may disappear by themselves. This condition often is related to sleep problems, poor conditioning, or an old injury. In fact, fibromyalgia is a chronic disorder characterized by widespread musculoskeletal pain, fatigue and tenderness in localized areas of the neck, spine, shoulders, and hips called "tender points."

People with this syndrome may also experience sleep disturbances, morning stiffness, irritable bowel syndrome, anxiety and other symptoms. It primarily occurs in women of childbearing age, but children, the elderly and men may also be affected.

Although the cause of fibromyalgia is unknown, some scientists believe that an injury or trauma may cause the syndrome. This injury may affect the central nervous system. Fibromyalgia may be associated with changes in muscle metabolism, such as decreased blood flow, causing fatigue and decreased strength. Others believe an infectious agent, such as a virus in susceptible people, may trigger the syndrome, but no such agent has been identified.

Fibromyalgia is difficult to diagnose because many of the symptoms mimic those of other diseases. As per the criteria laid down a person is considered to have fibromyalgia if he or she has widespread pain for at least 3 months in combination with tenderness in at least 11 of 18 specific tender point sites.

Treatment of fibromyalgia requires a comprehensive approach. The physician, physiotherapist, and others in the medical support system, as well as the patient may all play an active role in the management of fibromyalgia. Studies have shown that aerobic exercise, such as swimming and walking, improves muscle fitness and reduces muscle pain and tenderness. Heat and massage may also give short-term relief. Antidepressant medications may help elevate mood, improve quality of sleep and relax muscles. Fibromyalgia patients may benefit ftom a combination of exercise, medication, physical therapy and relaxation.

Paget's Disease

This is a type of disorder in which the calcium in bones spreads unevenly. The bones most commonly affected are in the lower back, pelvis, tailbone, skull, and long bones of the legs. It is slightly more common in men than in women. It often begins between the ages of 50 and 70. Back pain may be a symptom, but most often there are no obvious symptoms. Paget's disease usually is discovered on a x-ray or bone scan done for reasons other than pain.

Food Poisoning and Reiter's Syndrome

Food or water spoiled by salmonella or certain other bacteria can lead to a form of arthritis called Reiter's Syndrome. People who develop this rare kind of arthritis seem to have a defect in their body's defense system. This makes them more likely to develop arthritis in response to certain infections.

• • •

17

Ankylosing Spondylitis

This form of arthritis causes the joints in the spine to become stiff and swollen. In certain cases stiff joints can fuse (grow together). The most common symptoms are pain and stiffness in the buttocks and lower back (particularly in the morning) that continue for more than three months. Ankylosing spondylitis is most common in men and often begins between the ages of 20 and 40.

So it is clear that ankylosing spondylitis primarily affects the spine or back. The joints and ligaments that normally permit the spine to move become inflamed and stiff. The bones of the spine may grow together, causing the spine to become rigid and inflexible. Other joints such as the hips, shoulders, knees, or ankles also may become involved. Heredity seems to play a role in determining who gets ankylosing spondylitis as it is noticed that approximately one in five people affected by ankylosing spondylitis have a relative with the same disorder. A gene called HLA-B27 is present in over 90 percent of people with ankylosing spondylitis. Ten to fifteen percent of individuals who inherit the gene will demonstrate ankylosing spondylitis.

Almost all people with ankylosing spondylitis can expect to lead normal and productive lives. Despite the chronic nature of the illness, only a few people with ankylosing spondylitis will become severely disabled. The management of pain and the control of inflammation can reduce the daily problems that may occur with ankylosing spondylitis. By correct posture and almost always involved body position and by doing exercises daily, the individual can control many of the effects of the disease.

Symptoms of ankylosing spondylitis appear most frequently in young men between the ages of 16 and 35. It is less common in women, whose symptoms are often milder and more difficult to diagnose. About five percent of ankylosing spondylitis begins in childhood; boys are more likely to have it than girls.

When children develop ankylosing spondylitis, it usually begins in the hips, knees and bottoms of heels or big toes and may later progress to involve the spine. The inflammation in ankylosing spondylitis usually starts with the back pain. Typically, symptoms lessen with movement and exercise. Over a period of time, pain and stiffness may progress into the upper spine and even into the chest and neck. Ultimately, the inflammation can cause the sacroiliac and vertebral bones to whole spine become rigid. Similarly, the bones in the chest may fuse, causing a loss of normal chest expansion when breathing. The hips, shoulders, knees or ankles also may become inflamed and painful and eventually lose their mobility. The heels may become affected, making it uncomfortable to stand or walk on hard surfaces. Ankylosing spondylitis is a systemic disease, meaning it affects the entire body in some people. It can cause fever, loss of appetite and fatigue and it can damage other organs besides the joints, such as the lungs, heart and eyes.

The eye is the most common organ affected by ankylosing spondylitis. Eye inflammation (iritis) occurs from time to time in one fourth of people with ankylosing spondylitis. Iritis results in a red, painful eye that worsens by looking at bright light. It is a serious condition requiring immediate medical attention by an ophthalmologist. Less frequently, ankylosing spondylitis may be associated with a scaly skin condition called psoriasis. In rare cases, ankylosing spondylitis may cause problems with the heart, lungs, or intestines. Symptoms similar to that seen in ankylosing spondylitis also may occur along with such conditions as psoriasis, inflammatory bowel disease, or Reiter's syndrome. Doctors usually base their diagnosis of ankylosing spondylitis on symptoms (pain, stiffness) and x -rays showing involvement of the sacroiliac joint at the back of the pelvis. If the symptoms and x-rays suggest ankylosing spondylitis, but the diagnosis is uncertain, the doctor may perform a blood test to check you for the HLA - B27 gene. About 90 percent of people diagnosed with ankylosing spondylitis do test positive for this gene. Treatment for ankylosing spondylitis should be, designed to reduce pain and stiffness, prevent deformities and maintain the normal activities.

• • •

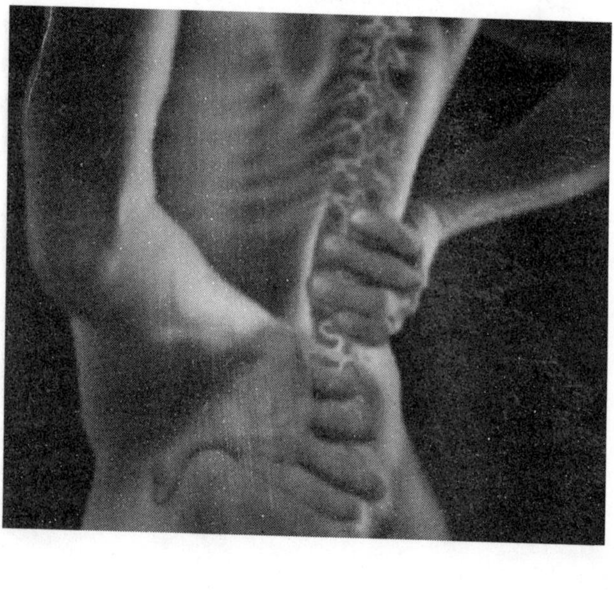

18

Back Pain Causes / Symptoms / Investigations

Back, having so many parts, makes easy to develop a problem into itself. Anything that puts pressure on the back muscles or nerves can cause pain. Any illness or damage to the spine also can cause pain. The cause of most acute back pain is unknown, but probably is due to minor strains, sprains, and overuse. Emotional stress may add to the pain, especially since it slows the rate of recovery. Other possible causes of back pain include a ruptured intervertebral disc, spinal stenosis, osteoarthritis, anykylosing spondylitis, an injury or accident, rheumatic-related problems or other conditions.

Many of the problems that cause back pain are the result of injury and degeneration of the intervertebral disc. Degeneration is a process where wear and tear causes deterioration. The disc is subjected to different types of stress as we use our backs each day. Bending over results in compression of the disc and may also cause the disc to bulge backwards towards the spinal canal and nerves. The facet joints must also shift to allow the bending to occur. Twisting and bending together is perhaps the greatest stress on the parts of the spine, especially the disc.

Probably, the earliest of changes that occur in the disc are tears in the annulus portion of the intervertebral disc. The annulus is a large round ligament and the tears in the annulus heal the same way as the tears in other ligaments do, that is by scar formation. Scar tissue is not as strong as normal tissue. The repeated cycle of many annular tears healing by scar tissue leads to the disc that finally begins to degenerate.

What happens when the Disc begins to Degenerate?

As the degeneration of the disc progresses the nucleus pulposus loses some of its water content. It becomes stiff and loses the ability to act as a shock absorber. The process may continue until the disc is collapsed. Bone spurs may form as the body's response to this degeneration. These spurs are thought to be the result of excess motion at the spinal segment. Eventually, bone spurs form around the nerves of the spine as well.

One of the most dramatic injuries to the lumbar spine is the Herniated Disc. In this injury, a tear in the annular ligament allows the nucleus pulposus to squeeze into the spinal canal. If the disc material compresses the nerve root, there is pain, numbness, and weakness in the areas supplied by the nerve. There is a considerable amount of evidence to suggest that it's not only the pressure that plays a part in the symptoms from a herniated disc. The nucleus material that is squeezed out against the nerve seems to set up an inflammatory response in the nerves causing pain.

Symptoms

Low back pain can be divided into two main types:

- Mechanical Type pain
- Compressive Type pain

Mechanical type back pain results from inflammation caused by irritation or injury to the disc, the facet joints the ligaments or the muscles of the back. A common cause of mechanical pain is disc degeneration. A typical muscle strain, or lumbar strain, can also be the cause of mechanical type symptoms. Mechanical type back pain usually starts near the lower spine. Mechanical type pain may also spread to include the buttock and thigh areas. It rarely extends below the knee.

Compressive or neurogenic (meaning nerve related) type pain occurs when the nerve roots that leave the spine are irritated or pinched. A common cause of compressive pain is a herniated disc. The nerves that leave the lower lumbar spine join to form the sciatic nerve. This nerve provides sensation and controls the muscles of the lower leg. Pressure or irritations on the nerve roots of the lumbar spine that come together to form the sciatic nerve can interfere with the normal function of the sciatic nerve. One of the earliest signs of pressure on a nerve root is numbness in the area supplied by the nerve. Pain is commonly felt in the same area, usually extending below the knee to the foot. In cases where there is pressure on a nerve root as it comes out of the spine, it is not unusual for the back itself to be painless. This can be confusing at times since there is no back pain but the problem is located in the lumbar spine. Finally, the muscles that the nerve controls may become weak and the reflexes may disappear. This is because the pressure on the nerve roots interferes with the signals from the brain to the muscles. There is no signal going from the brain to the muscle to tell it to contract.

Spinal stenosis can also cause compressive type pain. In some people, degeneration of the spine can result in a narrowing of the spinal canal- the bony tube where the spinal nerves are located. This causes all of the nerves within the spinal canal to become inflamed, and fail to work properly. One problem that occurs when the tube is too small, is that the nerves cannot get enough blood supply to work properly. The nerves may be normal when the body is at rest, but once it is active the nerves need more blood flow to get more oxygen. If the tube is too tight, the blood supply cannot increase. One of the symptoms of this cause is numbness. It may be in one or both the legs. The numbness may become worse with activities. The pain can involve both of the lower extremities. The pain becomes worse on walking and gets better after short periods of rest. Weakness of the muscles of both legs may also occur, and again, this may get worse when activity increases.

In very few cases, a disc herniation can be so big that it fills the entire spinal canal. The immediate pressure on the nerves in the spine may cause paralysis of the muscles that control the bowels and bladder. When the control over the bowels or bladder is lost, it is better to contact the physician immediately. **If the back pain is accompanied by any of the following, the doctor should be consulted:**

- weakness or numbness in one or both legs
- pain going down one leg below the knee
- back pain from a fall or injury
- back pain accompanied by fever
- pain that continues to interrupt sleep after three nights
- back pain that remains after six weeks of home treatment

Diagnosis

To enable the doctor to diagnose the problem correctly the complete history of the back pain should be provided. The doctor may ask a number of questions as listed below:

- What are the symptoms?
- What kinds of aches or pains?
- Where exactly is the pain?
- Where is the pain the most severe?
- When did the pain begin?

- How long it lasts?
- Did-something specific cause the back pain, such as an accident or injury?
- What home treatments is undertaken?
- Was there any additional stress when the pain began ?
- Is there any other health problems?
- What kind of work does the patient do?
- Types of recreational activities in which the patient participates

Next, the doctor will make a clinical/physical examination. During the exam, **the doctor may perform any of the following:**

- observe the muscles and joints
- ask to sit and lie down
- ask to move the back in different positions
- observe the most painful area
- check if other areas of the body are tender or painful (such as the kidneys, intestines, or other organs).

If the doctor can identify the likely cause of the back pain, at this point, no further tests will be needed. If the doctor needs more specific information, the following tests may be advised:

X-RAY

Studies show that in many cases of routine back pain, x - rays may not initially be necessary. However, the signs and symptoms will determine what type of study should be done. In certain cases, x-rays might indicate that the pain is due to:

- injury in one or more of the back bones
- a tumour in the spine
- a deformity in the spine
- ankylosing spondylitis

CAT Scan (Computerized Axial Tomography)

Only a few people with lower back pain need a CAT scan. If the doctor advises one, a special machine takes an x-ray scan of the area. A computer turns this scan into a three-dimensional view of the back. This helps the doctor see if there is a ruptured disc that can't be seen on regular x-rays; CAT scan also helps in detecting spinal stenosis, tumours and infections of the spinal cord.

MRI (Magnetic Resonance Imaging)

MRI is another way to make very clear pictures of parts of the spine. The MRI does not use x -rays or radioactive dyes. It can provide clearer pictures of soft tissues such as muscles, cartilage, ligaments, tendons and blood vessels in addition to bone structure. To take a MRI picture, the body must be moved very slowly through a tube in the centre of the machine, which contains very powerful magnets. People, who are claustrophobic or whose bodies contain certain kinds of metal objects, may not be able to tolerate the procedure.

The MRI scanner shows the nerves and disc quite clearly. No special dyes or needles are necessary. The MRI scan is, perhaps, too good at showing the anatomic details of the spine. There is a growing body of evidence that suggests that not all abnormalities that show up on the MRI scan are really the cause of the individual patient's problem related to back pain. Abnormalities, such as bulging discs, show up frequently in normal persons who have never had any problem with their back. Hence, it should be kept in mind that a MRI scan is a great test to show the lumbar spine anatomy and it must be correlated carefully with the symptoms so that the findings aren't blown out of proportion.

Type of Back Pain

Back pain may be acute (generally severe, but short-lived), subacute or chronic (long-lasting or occurring often).

Acute Back Pain

- Pain usually lasts from one to seven days.
- Pain may be mild or severe.
- An accident or injury occasionally may cause pain.
- About 80 percent of all back pain are acute.

Subacute Back Pain

- Pain usually lasts from seven days to seven weeks.
- Pain usually is mild and occasionally severe.
- Pain generally is unrelated to other illness.
- About 10 to 20 percent of all back pain are subacute.

Chronic Back Pain

- Pain usually lasts more than three months.
- Pain may be mild or severe.
- Pain may be related to other illness or may have no identifiable cause.
- About five to 10 percent of all back pain is chronic.

Structure of Back

The back is held upright by muscles attached to the backbone. Doctors often refer to the backbone as the spine, spinal column, or backbone and find the discs located between each vertebra. These discs are made of cartilage, which is a soft, elastic material, Discs act as cushions, or shock absorbers. Their main job is to protect the joints from wearing out. Most joints contain a slippery substance called synovial fluid that keeps them moving smoothly.

The spinal cord is very important because it transmits electrical signals between the brain and the nerves in the legs, arms, back and other parts of the body. The spinal cord runs through a hole in each vertebra of the upper and middle parts of the backbone, much like a piece of string through a beaded necklace. The space it runs through is called the spinal canal. At times, a message might pain or discomfort. The pain signal is an important one, because it tells that some part of the body needs attention.

A serious injury to the neck or upper back runs the risk of damaging the spinal cord, causing paralysis of the parts of the body below the injury. It should be noted that the spinal cord is not present in the lower part of the backbone. Here the spinal canal contains a sack of nerves, the cauda equina. The backbone, with all its parts, cannot hold itself upright. It needs strong muscles, tendons, and ligaments for support. Muscles help to move or hold the position. Tendons fasten muscles to bones, and ligaments stretch from one bone to another to hold bones together.

Myelogram

During a myelogram, a special liquid dye called contrast medium is injected into the spinal canal then X-rays are taken of the area. The contrast medium can make problem areas show up more clearly on the x-ray. A myelogram may be ordered to detect problems such as spinal stenosis or spinal cord tumours. If surgery is being considered, particularly for a person who has had a serious back injury, many neurosurgeons will require a myelogram beforehand.

Bone Scan

During a bone scan, a very small amount of radioactive liquid is injected into a vein which concentrates in the bones for a short time. A special radioactive detecting machine scans the area of concern to produce a picture. Occasionally bone scans are done to look for damage or tumours in the bones themselves. However, back pain is rarely due to diseases of the bones.

Electrodiagnostic Studies

Electrodiagnostic studies are used to help confirm the presence of nerve compression in the spine. An electrodiagnostic study consists of two tests. One is an electrical test, which is designed to study nerve conduction. In this test the nerve is given an electrical stimulation, and the speed of the impulse is measured. The other test is a needle test called an electromyogram, or EMG. The purpose of this test is to study the muscles for primary disease or for the effect of nerve compression on the muscle. The compression is especially seen in herniated discs or spinal stenosis.

Blood Tests

If the doctor orders blood tests, a laboratory technician will carefully draw a small amount of blood from a vein in the arm, which will be tested in the laboratory. Anyone of the following blood tests may be advised:

- erythrocyte sedimentation rate (sed rate)
- haematocrit and haemoglobin
- white blood cell count
- HLA B-27 test
- chemical profile (SMAC)

Treatment

The treatment of back pain ranges from simple reassurance that nothing is wrong to extremely delicate surgery. Each case is different and treatment must be individualized to meet the circumstances. Treatment falls into two major categories:

- Conservative treatment - which includes exercise, medications, physical therapy and other non-operative therapy.
- Surgical treatment - which includes laminectomy, diskectomy and spinal fusion in selected conditions.
- Treatment for any back condition should involve two goals:
- To relieve the immediate problem
- To reduce the risk of re-injury

Exercise plays an important role in achieving both of these goals.

More than 85 percent of people with lower back pain improve with minimal treatment in a matter of days. However, if back problems persist, doctors generally prescribe one or more of the following treatments. For some back conditions, the doctor may refer the patient to another specialist such as an orthopedist, rheumatologists; physical or occupational therapist, psychologist, psychiatrist or surgeon.

Rest

The most common treatment doctors recommend for severe back pain is bed rest. Different people require different amounts of rest. Usually, two to three days of staying in bed, except to go to the bathroom, will be enough to ease the back pain. The doctor may be consulted to know if special pillows or devices are necessary to give additional support to the neck, back, or feet.

Heat and Cold

Many people have found that hot and cold treatments help relieve back pain. It is advisable to try both to find out which of the two works best.

Heat relaxes muscles and soothes painful areas. There are many ways to apply heat. Some people like hot showers or baths, while others prefer using heat lamps, heating pads or warm compresses. For the persons having arthritis, heating the muscles first might make it easier to do back exercises. Care should be taken not to fall asleep while using heat.

Cold has a numbing effect. This often helps relieve pain. One of the following methods may be tried for applying cold:

- an ice bag
- a large ice cube used to massage the area
- frozen package of vegetables (peas work best)
- a commercially made cold pack. Be sure not to leave ice on after the skin becomes numb as this could lead to localized frostbite. Persons sensitive to ice or having decreased circulation or sensation should not use cold treatment.

• • •

19

Medication and Surgery of Back Pain

If the back pain is not relieved using other forms of treatment, the doctor may prescribe medication. The choice of medication depends on the back pain. For example, medications called analgesics can relieve pain. Other medications called muscle relaxants can help relax tight muscles. If the back pain is caused by arthritis, the doctor can prescribe medication that reduces inflammation as well as relieve the back pain. The most common medications prescribed are called Nonsteroidal anti-inflammatory drugs (NSAIDs). Aspirin and ibuprofen are NSAIDs. Some other NSAID medicines are also prescribed when needed.

Some medications are highly addictive. Pain medication used for prolonged periods has the potential of leading to addiction. No medication will cure back pain of degenerative origin. Medications are used to control pain, inflammation, muscle spasm, and sleep disturbance. Many physicians feel that narcotic medications should not be used on a continuous basis to treat chronic low back pain. There are certain circumstances where pain management specialists are finding that chronic narcotics will actually benefit certain groups of patients with chronic low back pain, but the majority of low back pain will not require this approach.

If simple measures fail to control the back pain, an Epidural Steroid Injection (ESI) may be suggested. The epidural steroid injection involves placing a small amount of cortisone into the bony spinal canal. Cortisone is a very powerful anti-inflammatory drug that may bring the inflammation surrounding the nerves under control and ease the pain. The epidural steroid injection is not always successful. These injections are reserved for cases where all other conservative measures have failed or as a last attempt to postpone surgery.

A patient should be well informed about his medication and should clarify all doubts regarding the medicines from the doctor.

About Medication

- What will the medication do?
- How long will it take to show results?
- What is the name of the medication?
- Is there a generic brand?
- Are there any side effects?
- How should the medication be taken?
  (i.e. before or after meals, with or without food, etc.)
- How often the medication is to be taken?
- What is to be done if the dose is not taken at the specified time?

The doctor should be told about the other medication that has been taken as sometimes certain medications cannot be taken together.

Surgery

People with sciatica or spinal stenosis often benefit from surgery. A few people with tumors within the spinal canal require it. Other than that, few people with back pain need surgery. Most people can be treated successfully with rest, exercise, and medication. Surgery does not always work for many common kinds of back pain, and it is difficult to know who will be helped and who will not. An orthopedist or neurosurgeon can help to decide if a back operation is necessary. It is always recommended to seek a second opinion.

If surgery is suggested for a problem, the best operation for that specific problem will be suggested. Although back surgery is not so common in India, so many people have back problems at some time in their lives that there are substantial number of back operations done. However, the vast majority of people with back problems never have back surgery and function quite well with a minimal effect on their daily lives. An overview of the general types of back surgery that are sometimes necessary is given below.

One of the most common surgical procedures is a diskectomy, the removal of a herniated disc to relieve pressure on a nerve root. The first step is to remove a portion of the lamina of the vertebra. The lamina is the portion of the vertebra that forms the roof over the spinal nerves. Removing a portion of the lamina creates a window into the spine. The nerves are then pulled to the side so that the herniated disc can be seen. Small instruments are then used to remove the herniated disc material. Most of the nucleus pulposus is removed to prevent the disc from herniating again. Once the disc material is removed, the nerves are free of pressure and irritation. The lamina and the area of the disc that is removed fill with scar tissue very rapidly.

When the major problem appears to be spinal stenosis the spinal canal needs to be made larger. This is done by performing a complete laminectomy. The lamina is the backportion of the spine and forms the upper portion of the spinal canal. The term laminectomy means to remove the lamina. Removal of lamina allows more room for the nerves and enables the surgeon to remove bone spurs around the nerves. This allows more room for the nerves of the spine and reduces the irritation and inflammation on the spinal nerves. The bone does not grow back. Instead, scar tissue replaces the lamina and protects the spinal nerves.

If the back problem is the result of segmental instability, a spinal fusion may be suggested. A spinal fusion involves placing a bone graft between two or more vertebrae, causing the vertebrae to grow together or fuse. The bone graft is usually taken from the bones of the pelvis at the time of surgery. There are two general types of spinal fusion:

- Posterior fusion
- Interbody fusion

In the posterior fusion, the bone graft is placed on the back side of the vertebrae. During the healing process the vertebrae then fuse, or grow together. This creates a solid block of bone between the vertebrae, and the vertebra that is fused together act like one bone. The Interbody fusion differs by placing the bone graft between the vertebrae, where the disc has been removed. Once again, the healing process causes the vertelirae to fuse, creating a solid block of bone between the fused vertebrae. Both fusions accomplish the same thing. The vertebrae grow together, or fuse into one bone. The goal of a spinal fusion is to stop the motion between two vertebrae that comes from segmental instability. Fusing the vertebrae together reduces the mechanical back pain and impingement on the nerve root that comes from too much motion between the vertebrae.

• • •

20

Backache Top 10 Advices

1. Take over the counter painkillers. But be cautious. A recent study found that regular use of common pain relieved such as Ibuprofen may cause high blood pressure.
2. See an osteopath or chiropractor for manipulation of the spine and exercises. You will require between two and six sessions.
3. Try acupuncture, in which very thin needles are inserted under the skin.

   Pain relief can result from the release of endorphins, the body's own pain relieving chemicals.
4. See your GP, who may prescribe stronger anti inflammatory pain killers than can be bought over the counter.

   Nonsteroid anti-inflammatories can have side effects, including ulcers.
5. Your GP may also prescribe a muscle relaxant such as diazepam, to be taken for a short period to reduce muscle spasms.
6. Have physiotherapy. A physiotherapist can design an exercise programme to improve your flexibility, strengthen your back and improve your posture.

7. Take oral steroids, which may be prescribed during episodes of pain. These reduce inflammation in the spine. Oral steroids are intended for use for short periods of time
8. Have steroid injections, which can reduce pain and inflammation.
9. Have an epidural. Corticosteroid drugs can be injected into the spine and are used in the treatment of sciatica. The effects will last a few months.
10. Have surgery- usually the last resort and only in the most severe cases. Back operations include spinal fusion and the removal of disc material that is compressing nerves.

Novel Spinal Surgery

Scientists in the US are using a novel technique to remove tumours from the cervical region of the spine that were previously thought inoperable, according to a study published in operative Neurosurgery.

Called a lateral paramedian transpedicular approach, the technique uses standard and innovative devices to first remove and then reconstruct portions of the cervical spine.

Once the bone is removed, surgeons have a direct line of sight to the tumour and can remove it in entirety without a touch to the spinal cord.

• • •

21

Proper Exercises & Postures for Backache

For many people, the key to a healthy back is proper exercise. Some exercises are designed to strengthen the back and stomach muscles, while other exercises are designed to improve the posture. A 30-minute aerobic programme, three times a week, is ideal for overall fitness. Walking and or water exercises are highly recommended for most people with back problems. The right kind of exercise programme may help keep the back problem under control. It makes easy to continue the daily activities.

In the early stages, when the back is still quite painful, the specific exercises, which reduce the pain are advised. These exercises are helpful in easing pain through relaxation. The positioning exercises help in placing the spine at a resting position. These exercises give relief to sore muscles and joints.

Movement is also important, even when the back is still painful. The therapists suggest careful movements that can safely ease pain by providing nutrition and lubrication to injured areas. Movement of joints and muscles also signals the nervous system to block incoming pain. As the back becomes less painful, the exercises will be changed to focus on improving the overall health of the back. These changes will focus on:

- flexibility
- strength
- coordination

- aerobic conditioning

Exercises help in reducing pain and to keep the spine in the neutral position. Tight muscles can cause an imbalance in spinal movements and make the risk of injury to these structures more likely. Flexibility exercises for the trunk and lower limbs are helpful in establishing a pattern of safe movement. The stretching exercises also increase the flexibility in the muscles and ligaments of the back and reduce the chance of re-injury.

The next stage of exercise focuses on the strength of the muscles that support the spine. These muscles help bring the spine into the normal shape. Well-trained abdominal, back and hip muscles can help hold the back in a neutral position, almost forming a natural corset. Strength training is simple to do at home and doesn't require any expensive equipment.

Posture exercises help train the muscles in the right movements between the pelvis and low back. Learning how to find and hold the neutral position of the spine - is the key for a safe and healthy posture. It should always be kept in mind that the position of the pelvis determines the curve in the low back. Forward rotation increases the curve while the backward rotation straightens the curve. By practicing these exercises one will become more comfortable in using the neutral spine position in the daily activities. Strong muscles need to be coordinated. As the strength of the spinal muscle increases, it becomes important to train those muscles to work together.

Learning any physical activity requires practice. Muscles must be trained so that the physical activity should always remain under control. Muscles trained to control safe movement of the spine reduce the chance of injury. There are certain exercises that train the back muscles to work together to protect the spine.

Finally, attention will be directed to increase the overall fitness. Muscles get the energy they need to work either by using oxygen to bum calories from the bloodstream or by burning sugars in the bloodstream quickly without using oxygen. By using oxygen, muscles are better able to move continuously, rather than in spurts. The word aerobic means intake of lot of oxygen. Fitness training, or aerobic training, conditions the muscles to become better able to obtain the nutrients and oxygen that they need from the blood. If muscles are more used to working in fits and spurts they are more likely to bum sugars without using oxygen. This is called anaerobic metabolism, and it doesn't work nearly as well as aerobic metabolism. As the muscles use up the nutrients and oxygen, they switch to anaerobic metabolism and chemical waste products are created that can cause pain in the muscles. Aerobic training increases the muscles ability to get rid of these waste products.

Exercise has other benefits as well. Exercise can cause chemicals called endorphins to be released into the blood. These chemical hormones act as natural pain relievers in reducing the pain. So, exercise can actually help control pain through the body's natural pain medication. It will be important to pick up an aerobic activity that is enjoyable and can be stuck to. But the exercise that makes the back pain worse should be avoided. The doctor or physical therapist may be consulted to know the right exercises.

Maintaining Good Posture

Mother Nature did not design the human spine to sit. Sitting, and especially sitting for long periods of time, is a lot harder on the back than lying down, standing up and even lifting (assuming that lifting is done properly).

This has something to do with what happens to the spine when the posture is changed from standing to sitting. The lower back has a natural curve called a lordotic curve. It's important to maintain natural lordosis. In this position, the structures that support the spine - the muscles, ligaments and discs can work in harmony.

If the back is not supported, the muscles will get very tired, very quickly. When this happens, the body slouches in an attempt to give those muscles a rest. The problem is that sitting in a slouched posture reduces the natured lumbar curve. That's one of the main reasons why so many people's discs bulge and/ or herniate.

By sitting properly in an ergonomically designed chair, the back will be supported correctly. But this may not be enough, as backs are not built to sit in the same position for long periods of time, even when the posture is perfect. Hence it is very important to practise techniques for good posture while sitting, standing or sleeping.

When Sitting

- Sit in a firm chair with armrests to relieve pressure in the back and shoulders.
- Keep the upper back straight and shoulders relaxed. Keep stomach muscles pulled in and maintain the proper curve in the lower back. Tightening the stomach and buttocks can do this. Some people are more comfortable sitting with the back of the chair at a 15 to 20 degree angle. A small cushion behind the lower back to maintain the natural curve of the back also can be quite helpful.
- Keep the knees slightly higher than the hips. Use a footstool or book under the feet if necessary.
- Keep the feet flat on the floor or other surface.
- Don't sit for a long period of time. Stand up every now and then so as to stretch tight muscles and give them a chance to relax.

When Standing

- Stand with weight equal on both feet.
- Avoid locking the knees.
- Ease tension in the back by placing one foot on a footstool.
- Those who stand for long periods of time should wear flat or low-heeled shoes.
- Keep the back straight by tightening the stomach muscles and buttocks.

When Sleeping

- Lie on the side with the knees bent.
- If feel more comfortable, place a pillow between the knees while sleeping on the side.
- If one sleeps on the back, ask the doctor or physical therapist if placing pillows under the knees would help the lower back pain or make it worse.
- Use a hard mattress.

Body Mechanics

Good body mechanics mean to keep good posture while in motion. For example, while lifting, the object lifted is to be held close to the body and lifting should be done with the weight on legs. Thus the normal back curves are maintained as the legs lift the load. Avoidance of twisting, particularly when carrying a load, is also important for good body mechanics.

- When bending down to lift an object, bend with the knees instead of the back.
- Hold the object close to you.
- Straighten the legs to lift the object.
- Get help with an object that is too heavy.

The type of shoes also affects the posture. High heels may put more stress on the lower back by changing the posture. It is more comfortable to wear low or flat heels. Cushion-soled shoes also provide "shock absorbency" for the spine.

WEIGHT LOSS

One way of reducing the back pain and improving the general health is to lose weight, preferably with a balanced diet along with regular exercise. Fad diets or fast weight-loss programs are to be avoided. These can be harmful and may cause new problems.

• • •

22

Cervical Spondylosis

What is the Cervical Spine

The cervical spine is made up of small circular bones (vertebrae) stacked on top of each other. Between each vertebrae is an intervertebral disc which acts like a shock absorber and allows flexibility of the spine. Muscles and ligaments run between, and are attached to, the vertebrae. Nerves from the spinal cord pass between the vertebrae going to the shoulder, neck, arm, and upper chest.

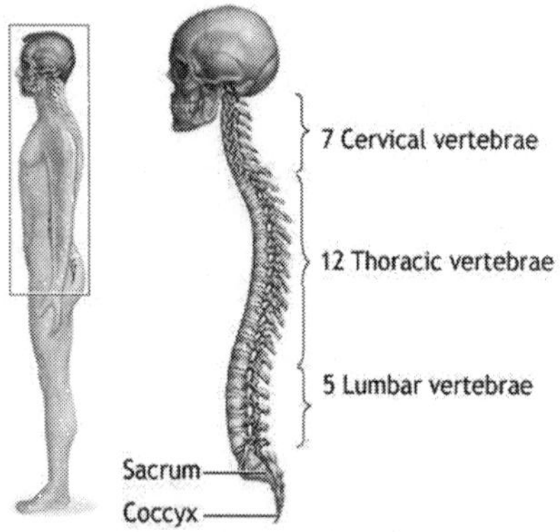

What is Cervical Spondylosis

To an extent, we all develop a degree of degeneration in the vertebrae and discs as we become older. However, cervical spondylosis is a term used if the degree of degeneration is more severe, and causes more symptoms, than is expected for a given age. As the 'discs' degenerate, over many years they become thinner. Sometimes the adjacent vertebrae develop small, rough areas of bone on their edges. The nearby muscles, ligaments, and nerves may become irritated by these degenerative changes which can cause troublesome symptoms.

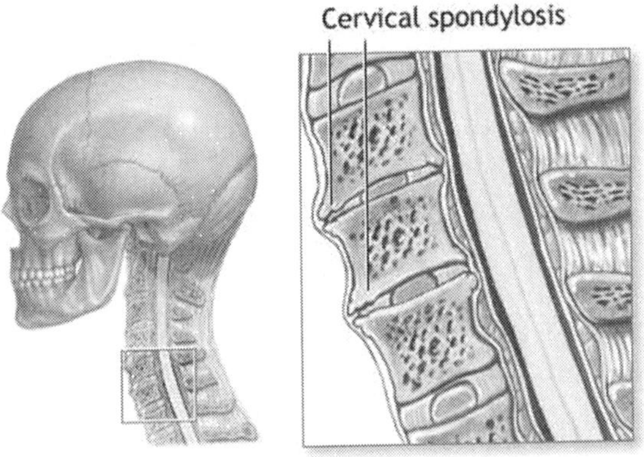

CAUSES

Cervical spondylosis is caused by chronic wearing away (degeneration) of the cervical spine, including the cushions between the neck vertebrae (cervical disks) and the joints between the bones of the cervical spine. There may be abnormal growths or "spurs" on the bones of the spine (vertebrae).

These changes can, over time, press down on (compress) one or more of the nerve roots. In advanced cases, the spinal cord becomes involved. This can affect not just the arms, but the legs as well.

The major risk factor is aging. By age 60, most women and men show signs of cervical spondylosis on x-ray. Other factors that can make a person more likely to develop spondylosis are:

- Past neck injury (often several years before)
- Severe arthritis
- Past spine surgery

Symptoms

Symptoms often develop slowly over time, but may start suddenly.

More common symptoms are:

- Neck pain (may radiate to the arms or shoulder)
- Neck stiffness that gets worse over time
- Loss of sensation or abnormal sensations in the shoulders, arms, or (rarely) legs
- Weakness of the arms or (rarely) legs
- Headaches, particularly in the back of the head

Less common symptoms are:

- Loss of balance
- Loss of control over the bladder or bowels (if spinal cord is compressed)

Exams and Tests

Examination often shows limited ability to bend the head toward the shoulder and rotate the head.

Weakness or loss of sensation can be signs of damage to specific nerve roots or to the spinal cord. Reflexes are often reduced.

The following tests may be done:

- CT scan or spine MRI
- Spine or neck x-ray
- EMG
- X-ray or CT scan after dye is injected into the spinal column (myelogram)

TREATMENT

Even if your neck pain does not go away completely, or it gets more painful at times, learning to take care of your back at home and prevent repeat episodes of your back pain can help you avoid surgery.

Symptoms from cervical spondylosis usually stabilize or get better with simple, conservative therapy, including:

- Nonsteroidal anti-inflammatory medications (NSAIDs)
- Narcotic medicine or muscle relaxants
- Physical therapy to learn exercises to do at home
- Cortisone injections to specific areas of the spine
- Various other medications to help with chronic pain, including phenytoin, carbamazepine, or tricyclic antidepressants such as amitriptyline

If the pain does not respond to these measures, or there is a loss of movement or feeling, surgery is considered. Surgery is done to relieve the pressure on the nerves or the spinal cord.

OUTLOOK (PROGNOSIS)

Most patients with cervical spondylosis will have some long-term symptoms. However, they respond to nonsurgical treatments and do not need surgery.

Possible Complications

- Chronic neck pain
- Inability to hold in feces (fecal incontinence) or urine (urinary incontinence)
- Progressive loss of muscle function or feeling
- Permanent disability (occasional)

WHEN TO CONTACT A MEDICAL PROFESSIONAL

Try home treatments, such as the use of a cervical collar (which you can buy at pharmacies) and over-the-counter pain medications.

Call your health care provider if:

- The condition becomes worse
- There are signs of complications
- You develop new symptoms (such as loss of movement or sensation in an area of the body).

Prevention

Many cases are not preventable. Preventing neck injury (such as by using proper equipment and techniques when playing sports) may reduce your risk.

Sex

Irvine et al defined the prevalence of ***cervical spondylotic*** myelopathy using radiographic evidence. In males, the prevalence was 13% in the third decade, increasing to nearly 100% by age 70 years. In females, the prevalence ranged from 5% in the fourth decade to 96% in women older than 70 years.

Homoeopathic Treatment

The most commonly used medicines used for the treatment of cervical spondylosis are..

Rhus Tox ..Pain and stiffness in the nape of the neck, pain between the shoulders,

Kalmia..pain from the neck down the arms, pain extending to the shoulder blades

Conium..cervical spondylosis with giddiness

Other commonly used medicines are:

Causticum,calcarea phos, calcarea flour, nux, hypericum

Note: Although I am giving the most commonly used medicines used for a particular complaint in my column it is advised that you consult a qualified homoeopathic doctor nearby to you and take his advise about the treatment of the problem.

Exercises & Yoga for Neck Pain and Spondylosis

Here are basic stretches and exercises that can be used by almost everyone in pain, though you should always consult your doctor before beginning an exercise plan. Take 10-15 minutes a day and go through the entire routine for maximum relief.

For each of the neck exercises, you should be seated comfortably with your shoulders, neck, and jaw as relaxed as possible.

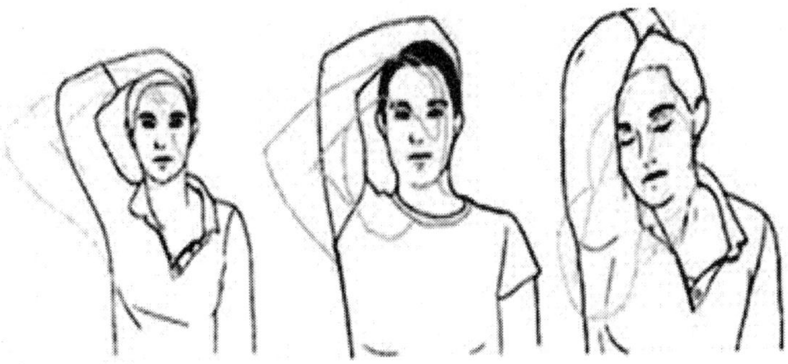

FIG 1 FIG 2 FIG 3

Reach your right arm over your head so that your palm is on top of your skull, your fingers resting just above the left ear. Allow the weight of your arm, along with light fingertip pressure, to gently bend the head toward your right shoulder (fig.1). Do not strain. Check to make sure your shoulders are still relaxed. You should be looking forward. Hold the pose for 30 seconds. Move your fingers toward the back left corner of your skull, this time allowing your head to bend forward and to the right, about 45 degrees in front of your shoulder (fig.2). Hold for 30 seconds. Now place your fingers at the back of your skull and gently pull your head straightforward, toward your chest (fig.3).

Hold for 30 seconds. Switch hands and repeat the stretches in reverse order: Pull forward, then 45 degrees in front of your left shoulder, and finally directly over your left shoulder. Do not push your head backward.

Do an isometric push against your hand to strengthen the neck. Hold your left palm against the left side of your head (fig.4). Push your left hand against your head while also pushing your head toward your left hand at about half strength. Hold for 30 seconds. Repeat with your right hand on the right side of the head. Do the same exercise, using either hand, with the back of the head (fig.5) and the forehead (fig.6).

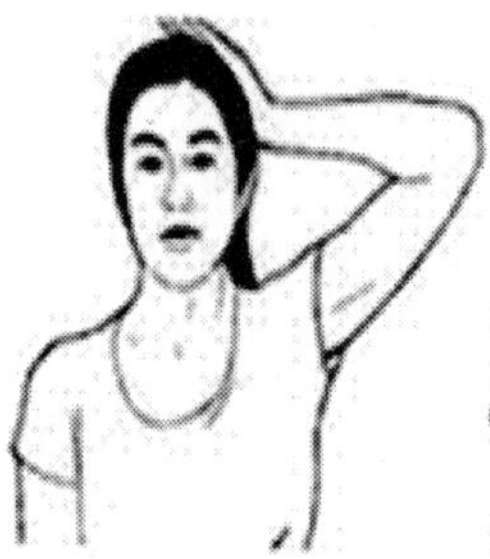

Fig 4

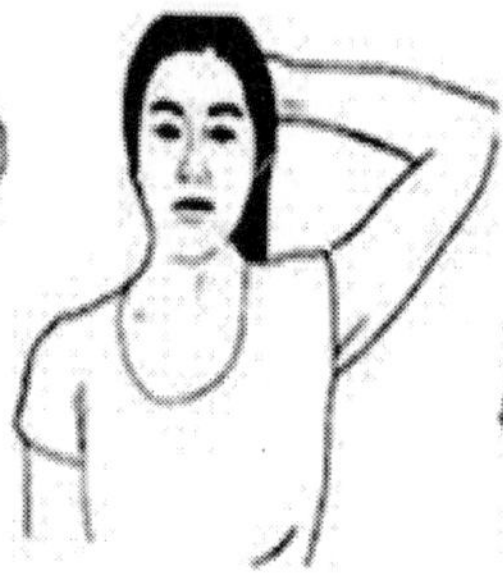

Fig 5

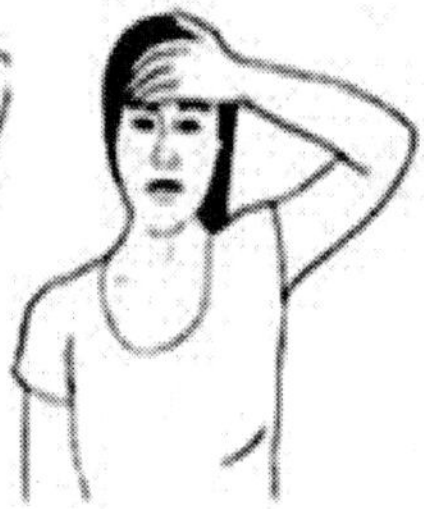

Fig 6

• • •

23

Yoga for Cervical Spondylosis and Chronic Neck Pain

If you determine you simply have a stiff neck, specific yoga exercises will help strengthen muscles and increase flexibility in the neck. Even gently exercising your neck helps lubricate and speed nutrients to the area. Here are a few exercises for your neck that are particularly helpful.

Neck Stretches

Follow these steps when practicing neck stretches:

- Start in seated position (cross legged)
- Sit up tall, reaching up through the top of the head
- Draw shoulders back
- Exhale, drop chin towards chest, keeping elbows and shoulders pulled back
- Inhale, raise the head back to centre
- Do this five times, then on the last exhale, drop the chin and stay in this position for three breaths, breathing through the nose
- Inhale, raise head back to centre
- Exhale, slowly drop right ear towards right shoulder
- Inhale, raise head back to centre
- Do this five times, then on the last exhale, drop the ear towards the right shoulder and stay in this position for 3 breaths

- Inhale, raise head back to centre
- Repeat on left side

If you continue to have a neck pain, your first task is to learn to re-establish a normal curve in as many situations as possible: sitting at your desk, standing in line at the grocery store, lying in bed.If done properly, all backward bends except Sethu Bandha Sarvangasana (Bridge Pose) engage your neck extensor muscles.

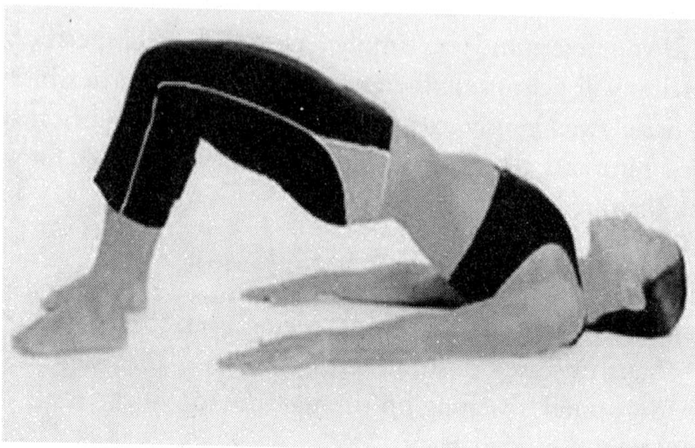

Backbend

Asanas like Salabhasana (Locust Pose) and Bhujangasana (Cobra Pose), backbends in which the weight of the head is lifted against gravity provide the most strengthening benefits for the back of the neck muscles. However, as you practice these asanas, see that you pull your shoulder blades away from your ears and do not to compress the back of your neck. Try to feel as if the cervical curve is distributed evenly throughout your entire neck and you're stretching your neck, even as you bend it backwards.

Neck strengthening exercises>

Bhujangasana (Cobra Pose)

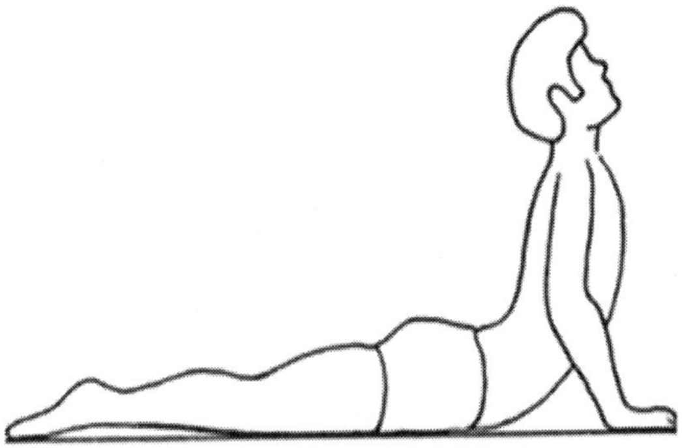

Cobra Posture (Bhujangasana)

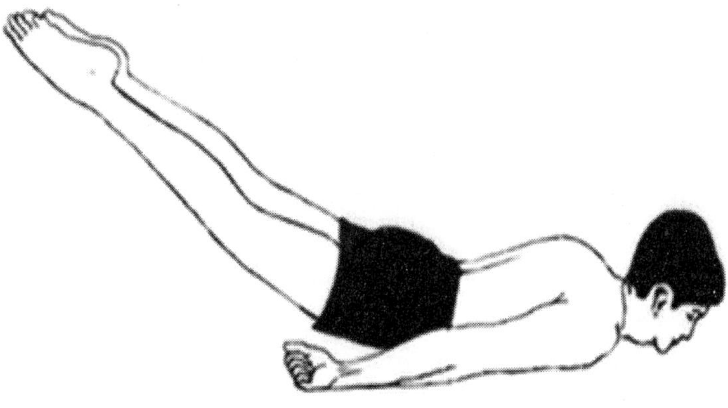

Locust Pose

Sarvangasana (Shoulderstand) can worsen the problem. As the pose drops your chin toward your chest, it makes it very easy to completely flatten the cervical curve or even curve the neck in the wrong direction. So, if you have a fairly recent, still painful, and acute neck injury like whiplash from an auto accident, avoid Shoulderstand. It would only exacerbate the injury, and practicing it too soon could significantly prolong your healing time.

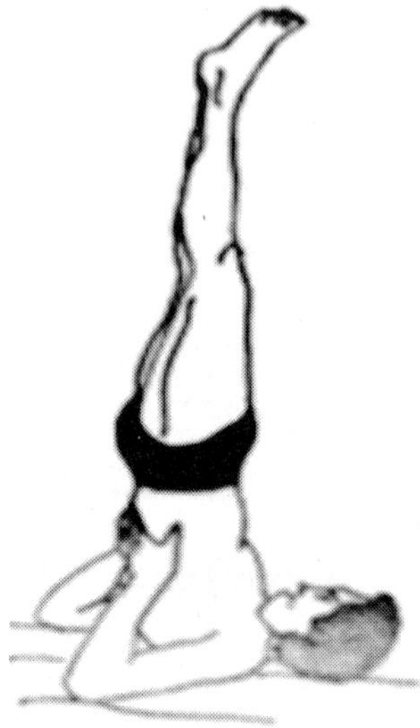

Shoulderstand (Sarvangasana)

HALF-CIRCLES

Half circles in the front can be done instead. To do this, first drop your chin to your chest. Move your chin towards the right shoulder then back to your chest. Then move your chin towards the left shoulder and back towards the chest. Repeat this movement three to five times.

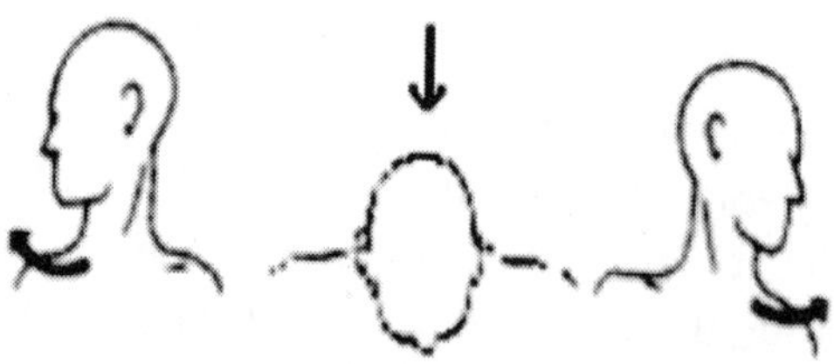

Clockwise and Anticlockwise Neck Rotation

Shoulder Moves

Hunch your shoulders as high as possible, then let them relax completely. Repeat this movement 5-6 times. Next, roll your shoulders in a backwards circular motion (lifting shoulders up, squeezing them back, dropping them down and then bringing them forward again). Repeat this motion 5-6 times, then move your shoulders in a forward circular motion. All these shoulder movements help to relax the muscles in your neck and upper back. Many of us hunch our shoulders unconsciously much of the time. Notice how they feel when they are relaxed and try to keep them this way.

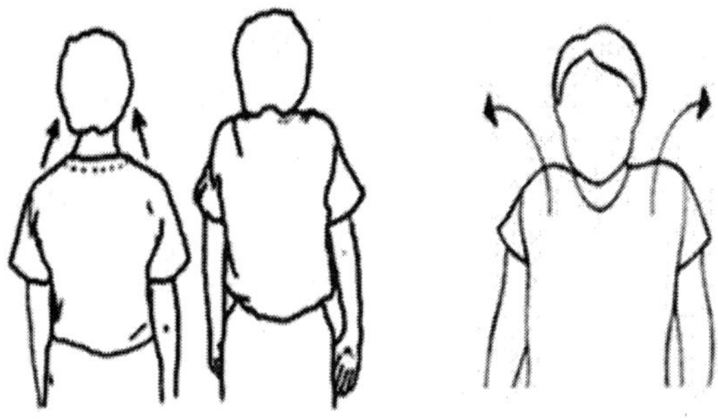

Hunch up the shoulders, roll back and bring to front. Drop down

Chest Expander

Stand up with your feet close together. Bring your hands behind your back and interlace your fingers. Tuck your tailbone in, so you don't arch your low back too much. As you inhale, lift your hands away from your tailbone. Squeeze your shoulder blades together and you lift your arms and stay in this position for 3-4 breaths. On your next exhale, lower your arms back down. This exercise helps strengthen the muscles in your upper back and relieve tension in your upper back and shoulders.

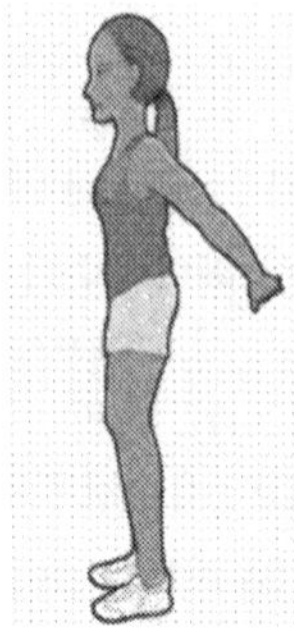

Arm Lift 1

ARM LIFTS

Bring your arms straight out in front of you with your palms facing each other. As you inhale, reach your arms overhead, bringing your arms next to your ears, if you can do so without any pain. As you exhale, bring your arms back down in front of you. Repeat 4-8 times. This helps to relieve tension and build strength in the muscles in the upper back.

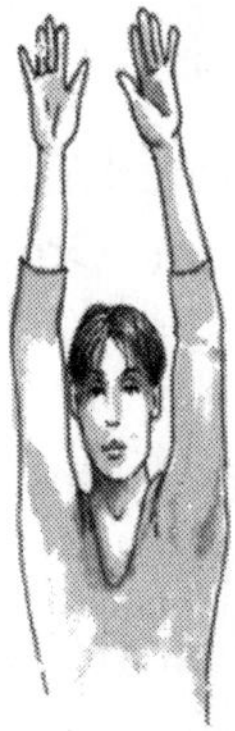

Arm Lift 2

PRESS IT

Place the palms of your hand against the back of your head and gently press while resisting with your head. Hold for a count of ten. Repeat with your palm on your forehead.

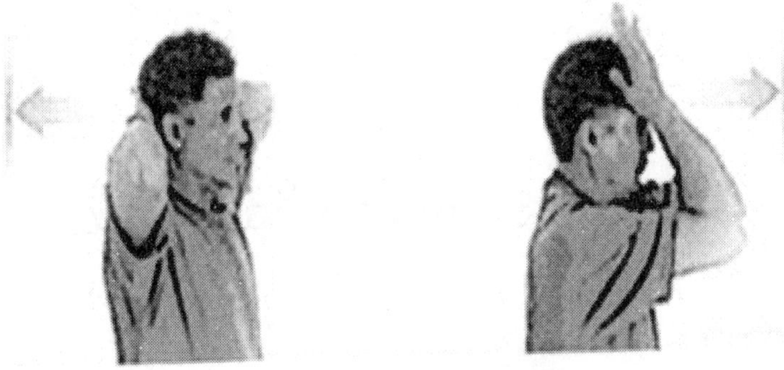

Pressing the neck against palm pressure

• • •

24

Compression of Spinal Cord

Injuries and disorders can put pressure on the spinal cord, causing back pain, tingling, muscle weakness, and other symptoms.

- The spinal cord may be compressed by bone, blood (hematomas), pus (abscesses), tumours, or a ruptured or herniated disk.
- Symptoms, such as back pain, abnormal sensations, muscle weakness, or impaired bladder and bowel control, may be mild or severe.
- Doctors base the diagnosis on symptoms and the results of a physical examination, magnetic resonance imaging (MRI), or another imaging test.
- Depending on the cause, surgery or a corticosteroid drug is used to relieve the pressure.

Normally, the spinal cord is protected by the spine, but certain injuries and disorders may put pressure (compress) on the spinal cord, disrupting its normal function. These injuries and disorders may also compress the roots of spinal nerves, which pass through the spaces between the back bones (vertebrae), or the bundle of nerves that extend downward from the spinal cord (cauda equina).

The spinal cord may be compressed suddenly, causing symptoms in minutes or over a few hours or days, or slowly, causing symptoms that worsen over many weeks or months.

CAUSES

The spinal cord may be compressed by the following:

- **Bone:** If the back bones (vertebrae) are broken (fractured), are dislocated, or grow abnormally (as occurs in cervical spondylosis), they may compress the spinal cord. Vertebrae that are weakened by cancer or osteoporosis may break after a slight or even no injury.
- **Connective tissue:** Connective tissue, such as ligaments, can compress the spinal cord after a severe spinal injury.
- **An accumulation of blood (hematoma):** Blood may accumulate in or around the spinal cord. The most common cause of a spinal hematoma is an injury, but many other conditions can cause hematomas. They include abnormal connections between blood vessels (arteriovenous malformations), tumours, bleeding disorders, and use of anticoagulants (which interfere with blood clotting) or thrombolytic drugs (which break up blood clots).
- **Tumours:** Cancer that has spread (metastasized) to the spine or the space around the spinal cord is a common cause of compression. Rarely, a tumour within the spine causes compression.
- **A localized collection of pus (abscess):** Less commonly, pus accumulates in or around the spinal cord and compresses it.
- **A ruptured or herniated disk:** A herniated disk can compress spinal nerve roots (the part of spinal nerves next to the spinal cord) and occasionally the spinal cord itself.

Sometimes the cauda equina syndrome results in compression of the spinal cord.

Sudden compression usually results from an injury, which often causes a fracture or dislocation of a vertebra. Gradual compression may result from cancer or cervical spondylosis, but bones weakened gradually (for example, by cancer or osteoporosis) may suddenly fracture, which can suddenly worsen compression (see Fractures: Compression Fractures of the Spine). Hematomas, abscesses, and ruptured disks can cause sudden compression but often cause compression gradually over days to weeks. The most common cause of slowly developing compression (over months to years) is cervical spondylosis (degeneration of disks and vertebrae in the neck—see Spinal Cord Disorders: Cervical Spondylosis).

What is the Cauda Equina Syndrome?

A bundle of nerves extends downward from the bottom of the spinal cord, through the lower vertebrae and over the sacrum (the bone at the base of the spine). This bundle is called the cauda equina, which means horse's tail in Latin, because that is what the bundle looks like. The cauda equina may be compressed by a ruptured or herniated disk, a tumour, an abscess, damage due to an injury, or swelling due to inflammation (as occurs in ankylosing spondylitis). The symptoms that result are called the cauda equina syndrome.

Pain is felt in the lower back, but sensation is reduced in the buttocks, thighs, bladder, and rectum—the area of the body that would touch a saddle. Thus, this condition is called saddle anesthesia. Sensation and muscle control may be impaired in the lower legs. Other symptoms may occur:

- Reduced sexual response, including erectile dysfunction in men
- Retention of urine
- Loss of bladder control (urinary incontinence)
- Loss of bowel control (fecal incontinence)
- Loss of reflexes in the ankle

People who have the cauda equina syndrome require immediate medical attention. Surgery to relieve the compression must be done as soon as possible. Corticosteroids may be given to reduce swelling.

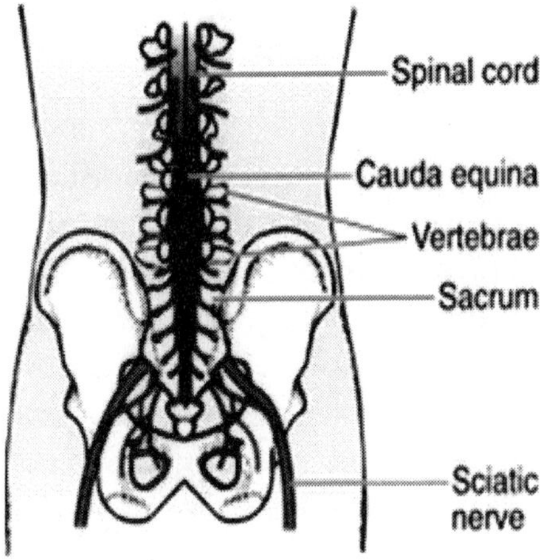

Symptoms

Slight compression may cause mild symptoms if it disrupts only some nerve impulses going up and down the spinal cord. These symptoms may include discomfort or pain in the back, slight muscle weakness, tingling, other changes in sensation, and, in men, difficulty initiating and maintaining an erection (erectile dysfunction). Pain may radiate down a leg, sometimes to the foot. If the cause is cancer, an abscess, or a hematoma, the back may be tender to the touch in the affected area. Sometimes sensation is lost. Reflexes, including the urge to urinate, may be exaggerated, sometimes causing muscle spasms and increased sweating. If compression increases, symptoms may worsen.

Substantial compression may block most nerve impulses, causing severe muscle weakness, numbness, retention of urine, and loss of bladder and bowel control. If all nerve impulses are blocked, paralysis and complete loss of sensation result. A beltlike band of discomfort may be felt at the level of spinal cord compression. Once compression begins to cause symptoms, the damage usually worsens from minimal to substantial unpredictably but rapidly in a few hours to a few days.

Diagnosis

People with symptoms suggesting spinal cord compression require immediate medical attention because prompt diagnosis and treatment may reverse or lessen loss of function.

Because the spinal cord is organized in a specific way, doctors can determine which part of the spinal cord is affected based on the symptoms and results of a physical examination. For example, if the legs (but not the arms) are weak and numb and bladder and bowel functions are impaired, the spine may be damaged at the midchest (thoracic) level. The location of pain or tenderness along the spine also helps doctors determine the site of the damage.

Magnetic resonance imaging (MRI) is done immediately. Or if MRI is unavailable, myelography (x-ray of the spinal column after injection of a radiopaque dye) with commuted tomography (CT) is done. These tests usually show where the spinal cord is compressed and may indicate the cause. MRI or myelography with CT scan detect a fracture or dislocation of a vertebra, a herniated disk, an abnormal bone growth, an area of bleeding, an abscess, or a tumour. During myelography, a spinal tap (lumbar puncture) is done to inject a small amount of radiopaque dye into the space around the cord. Thus, doctors can determine whether compression completely blocks the normal flow of cerebrospinal fluid through this space.

If the cause is thought to be a fracture or dislocation due to injury, x-rays may also be taken. They provide information quickly, enabling doctors to quickly evaluate the problem.

The cause of the compression is confirmed during surgery to relieve the pressure on the spinal cord.

If surgery is not done immediately and if MRI or myelography with CT detects an unidentifiable abnormal mass causing compression, a biopsy is done instead of surgery to identify it. Guided by CT, doctors insert a needle into the abnormal mass.

TREATMENT

If loss of function is partial or very recent (usually when compression occurs suddenly), the compression must be relieved immediately. When compression is detected and treated quickly, before nerve pathways are destroyed, treatment can prevent permanent damage to the spinal cord, and function is usually completely recovered. Surgery is typically needed to relieve compression. Surgery may also be needed to insert steel rods and thus stabilize the spine.

OTHER TREATMENT VARIES DEPENDING ON THE CAUSE.

For certain disorders, high doses of corticosteroids, such as dexamethasone or methylprednisolone, Some Trade Names MEDROL, are given intravenously as soon as possible. These disorders include tumours if the cause is unknown and possibly blunt injuries. Corticosteroids can reduce swelling in or around the spinal cord, which may be contributing to compression. If an abscess causes symptoms of spinal cord dysfunction (such as paralysis and loss of bowel or bladder control), a neurosurgeon surgically removes the abscess as soon as possible. Antibiotics are also given. If symptoms of spinal cord dysfunction have not developed, drawing the pus out through a needle, giving antibiotics, or both may be all that is needed.

If the cause is a hematoma, the accumulated blood is surgically drained immediately. People who have a bleeding disorder or who are taking anticoagulants are given injections of vitamin K and transfusions of plasma to eliminate or reduce the tendency to bleed.

If the cause is cancer, treatment usually includes surgery, radiation therapy, or both.

• • •

25

Pain in the Neck due to Blockage

We've all scoffed at that 'pain in the neck'. But watch out for that, especially after an accident- it could be a block in the neck artery and harbinger of a stroke. Clots cause 70-80% of all strokes and can cause paralysis and death in extreme cases.

Vivek Sharma, a 32 year old, was lucky. He was speeding in his car with a friend when severe pain hit the left side of his neck. Before his friend could react, Rahul slumped in his seat, unconscious. He was rushed to hospital where doctors gave him blood thinners to prevent further complications.

"This block in the neck artery," says Dr. V. K. Dixit, consultant, interventional neuro radiologist, VIMHANS, "usually happens during severe accidents or while doing head stands. The young are more susceptible to it due to their love of speed." Although any artery in the neck may be affected, internal carotid artery blockages are the most common.

Arteries are made of layers. Blockages generally occur between the first and second layers of an artery, says Dr Harsh Rastogi, interventional neuro radiologist, Apollo Hospital. "During an injury, there is a rent in the inner fragile layer of the artery. Blood with higher BP will rush in, making the vessel narrow and decreasing blood flow to brain. Before a full block occurs, this has to be treated with angioplasty and stenting to restore blood supply," he asserts.

The symptoms of a block include a "thunderclap" headache never experienced before, neck pain, vomiting and episodic blindness caused by decreased blood flow to the retina. "Usually the pain becomes severe over time," says Rastogi. "There might be loss of consciousness for a few seconds or sudden weakness which progresses over time, dizziness which does not respond to the usual medication, weakness in limbs and coma. These need urgent attention before a transient stroke occurs."

Studies have found that approximately 20% of strokes in the young are caused by carotid and vertebral artery blockages in the neck, compared to 2.5% in older patients. Annual incidence of carotid artery blockage in US is 2.6 per lakh population. In India, it's about 7-10 cases a month in any big hospital; 90% are trauma patients.

Dixit also warns of transient ischemic attacks (TIA)- temporary strokes where the patient recovers within 24 hours. Warning symptoms are weakness in one half of the body, temporary loss of speech and blurring of vision. "Just like an angina is an indication of heart attack, these are in dictions of a stroke coming on," he says.

Angioplasty reinforced with a stent can prevent a stroke from occurring. Here's how it works. Stents are compressed into a cathete. Using x-rays, an interventional neuro radiologist inserts the catheter through an incision in the groin. It's advanced through the femoral artery to tiny arteries where the clot busting drug is delivered directly into the hardened artery to break the clot.

The procedure costs between Rs. 1.5-2 lakh and the patient can often resume normal life with minimal or no after effects, say doctors.

• • •

26

Massage Step-By-Step for Relief of Pain in Different Organs

Just before you begin your massage check that your hands are clean and your nails fairly short with no jagged edges. Take off any rings if you wear them. You will find if you use aromatherapy oils regularly that your nails strengthen and your hands become smoother and more supple. Also, check with your massage partner to make sure there are no reasons to stop you going ahead.

The Feet

Probably the most neglected part of our bodies, feet deserve a loving massage from time to time. Make sure your partner is warm and comfortable. Uncover one foot by folding back the towel or blanket. Now pour a little of your chosen oil into the palm of one hand. Rub your hands together to evenly distribute the oil. Now you are ready to begin.

1. Enclose the foot between both hands (one on top, one underneath), then gently slide your hands off the foot coming forward to the toes. This movement should be slow and soothing. Repeat four or five times.
2. Gently circle around the ankles using your thumbs. This area can be tender, so go easy.
3. Rub over the top of the foot with your thumbs in little circles, coming down from the ankle area to the toes. Repeat three or four times.

4. Now rub each toe with the same little circular movements.
5. Rotate each toe twice in each direction.
6. Gently pull each toe between finger and thumb.
7. Zigzag down the sole of the foot from toes to heel with your thumbs overlapped.
8. Enclose the foot in your hands then rub them in opposite directions, to create frictions. This is very warming.
9. Hold the foot firmly and slowly rotate the ankle clockwise then anti-clockwise. Repeat a couple of times.
10. Repeat step 1.

Once complete, wrap the foot up again for warmth and repeat the movements on the other foot. By now your massage partner will be feeling more relaxed and at ease with your touch.

The Lower Legs And Knees

Warm a Little Oil in your Hands

1. With one hand behind the other, smooth the oil on to the front of the leg, starting at the top of the foot and working up to the knee. This movement distributes the oil and soothes and relaxes the whole area.
2. Rub across the front of the leg using both hands to create frictions. This increases the blood circulation to the area and reduces aches and pains.
3. Lift the leg up so the knee is bent. Squeeze and relax rhythmically down the muscles of the calf from knee to ankle. Repeat several times. Put the leg down.
4. Work around the kneecap in little circular motions with both hands. Be careful not to use too much pressure.
5. Now using your thumbs gently slide them around each side of the kneecap.

6. Stretch out your thumbs from your fingers to create an arch. Sweep over the whole knee using alternate hands several times.

Now wrap up the lower leg and proceed to the thigh.

The Upper Legs

1. Apply oil as for the lower leg.
2. Glide up the leg from knee to groin, using one hand behind the other. This movement should be fairly slow and rhythmical. Make sure your movements cover the whole of the thigh area. Repeat four to five times.
3. Stroke the upper inner thigh diagonally from knee to groin hand over hand. Repeat four or five times.
4. Squeeze and release rhythmically first along the inner thigh from knee to groin, then along the outer thigh.
5. Using your knuckles rake quickly up from the knee to the groin, taking in the whole thigh area. This is a friction movement and increases the surface blood circulation. You'll notice the skin colours quite quickly and feels warmer to the touch.
6. Uncover the lower leg, then effleurage the whole leg from foot to groin as in step 2.
7. Finish off by enclosing the foot in your hands a couple of times. Cover the leg then repeat all the movements on the other one.

By now you'll find your hands have become more sensitive to your partner and you'll notice differences in the skin texture and muscle tone.

The Hands and Arms

1. Smooth on the oil as before. When working on the arm it's easier to effleurage with one hand only, using the other to hold the arm steady.

2. Bend the arm at the elbow. Massage around the wrist with little thumb circles using both hands.
3. Work down from the wrist to the ends of the fingers using little thumb circles. Repeat five times.
4. Stretch each finger, then thumb, in turn between your finger and thumb.
5. Rotate the fingers and thumb first clockwise then anti-clockwise.
6. Turn the hand over and rub gently along the solar plexus (from centre wrist down the palm to the middle finger) using alternate thumbs. This is calming to the nervous system.
7. Rotate the hand at the wrist clockwise then anti-clockwise. To do this lock your fingers into your partner's.
8. Turn the hand over and work on the inside of the wrist up to the elbow using alternate sweeping movements. Repeat four or five times.
9. Bend the arm at the elbow and bring the lower arm up and across the chest. Squeeze all along the upper arm from elbow to shoulder using both hands.
10. Bring the arm back down to the side then effleurage the whole area from hand to shoulder four or five times. Cover the arm and repeat on the other side.

The Abdomen

The abdomen is a soft area protecting vital organs, so please be gentle. Fold the towel or blanket down to expose the area from just below the breasts to a couple of inches (centimetres) below the navel.

1. Apply oil, starting just under the rib-cage, working down and out towards the waist. Be careful to keep your hands

relaxed and contoured to your partner. Poking fingers feel very uncomfortable here.

2. With one hand on top of the other iron around the lower abdomen in large circles. Keep the pressure light and even.
3. Fan your hands out and work from the navel out to the waist. Slide your hands under the waist then gently pull them back round to the front again. Repeat several times.
4. Stroke diagonally with alternate hands from the waist down to below the navel, first on the left side, then on the right.
5. Stroke down from the solar plexus to the navel, one hand behind the other, to finish off this area.

The Backs of the Legs

1. Effleurage oil as for the front of the legs but working from the foot right up to the top of the thigh. Repeat four of five times.
2. Bend the leg at the knee, supporting it with one hand. Stroke firmly down the calf, across behind the knee, then back up to the foot several times keeping your hands contoured to the leg. Put the leg down.
3. Work up the calf to the knee, using little circles. Repeat several times to cover the whole calf.
4. Using your index and middle fingers, make small circular movements behind the knee. Be careful not to press too hard.
5. Squeeze rhythmically along the inner thigh from the knee upwards. Repeat on the outer thigh, doing each movement several times.
6. Diagonally stroke from the inner knee upwards and across the thigh. Repeat several times.
7. Finish by effleuraging the whole leg several times, from foot to thigh. Wrap up and repeat on the other leg.

The Back

Don't be at all surprised if your massage partner dozes off at this point. Back massage is extremely soothing and relaxing and great for relieving stress and tension.

Uncover the back to just show the buttock crease. At this point it is a good idea to place a small rolled-up towel under your partner's forehead otherwise he or she will have to turn his or her head sideways or end up with a squashed nose through which it is difficult to breathe.

1. Starting at the lower back effleurage oil using both hands. Work slowly up the back to the shoulders, pressing gently on the upward strokes, releasing the pressure as you come back down.
2. Starting at the base of the spine work up on either side, using gentle thumb pressure or little thumb circles. Repeat five or six times.
3. With reinforced hands (one on top of the other) sweep up the spine then work around the shoulder blades in a figure-of-eight movement. Repeat the figure-of-eight four or five times.
4. Now work around each shoulder blade individually, still with reinforced hands, in a circular motion. Repeat four of five times each side. You may feel knots (little bumps) around the shoulder blades. These are an indication of tension, and massage here gives great relief.
5. Work around the shoulder blades with your thumbs, helping to break down the knots and bumps. Allow your partner to be your guide as these areas can be tender.
6. Squeeze along the top of the shoulders from the neck out, using your fingers and thumbs. Repeat four to five times on each side.

7. Stroke up the back of the neck and out to the ears, using your thumbs.
8. Stand at your partner's head and sweep your hands down the centre back, across the top of the buttocks, then firmly pull up at the sides. Repeat five times.
9. Move to your partner's side and rub backwards and forwards over the whole back with frictions to warm the area.
10. Make thumb circles out from just above the buttock crease round towards the hips. This area can often be tender and massage here is soothing. Repeat several times.
11. Effleurage the whole back.
12. Gently stroke up the spine, hand over hand, several times, allowing your touch to get lighter and lighter.
13. Finish by gently holding your partner. Place one hand at the base of the spine, the other at the base of the neck. Hold this position and feel the warmth build up under your hands. After approximately one minute gently lift your hands off. Cover your partner over.

By now, he or she might be snoozing!

The Shoulders and Neck

If your partner is feeling very tense, and you haven't time to give a full body massage, working on the shoulders and neck will still offer great relief. For this your partner should be lying on his or her back. Uncover the chest by folding down the towel or blanket.

1. Apply oil to your partner's chest, shoulders and neck.
2. Begin effleuraging by placing both hands on the upper chest, fingers facing towards each other. Now, slowly pull your hands across the chest and out to the shoulders. Curve your hands round the shoulders and under them, then

bring your hands in to meet at the back of the neck. Stroke up the neck to the base of the skull, Repeat four or five times.

3. Gently knuckle the chest and shoulders in the sequence shown in the diagram on the left. To knuckle make your hands into relaxed fists, and move the knuckles in circular movements. This sounds more difficult than it is.
4. Gently turn your partner's head to one side. Stroke along the top of the shoulder and the side of the neck with your first three fingers. Repeat three times.
5. Repeat the above sequence, but circle your fingers this time. Do this three times.
6. Turn your partner's head to the other side and repeat movements 4 and 5. Return the head to the centre.
7. Slide your hands down your partner's back as far as you can comfortably reach. Find the groove each side of the spine with your fingers. Pull your hands up the spine with a little pressure on the groove each side. Repeat three times.
8. Now you are going to stretch the neck - these movements stretch out the muscles of the shoulders and ncek and ease tension. If your partner is relaxed you'll find you will take all the weight of the head. If he or she is tense, go easy and make the movements slow and gentle. You don't want any pulled muscles.
9. Cup both hands unde your partner's head, your fingers resting in the base of the skull. Lift the head slightly, then gently pull towards you. Lower the head slowly, then repeat.
10. Hold the back of the head in one hand and move it slowly towards the left shoulder while gently pressing down on the right shoulder with your other hand. Bring the head back to the centre and then repeat on the other side.
11. Finish with some effleurage movements as you begin.

The Face And Scalp

Until you've had the pleasurable experience of a face massage you probably won't have realized how much tension we hold in our faces. Think of frowning - this is caused by muscle action, and these musclcs tire just as much as those of any other part of the body. A caring face massage can smooth away some of this tension, leaving us looking (and feeling) more at ease and relaxed.

Offer to take your partner's hair off the face with a headband, as it will inevitably get a little only around the hairline during the massage. Be careful not to use too much oil on the face or you'll find it difficult to massage specific areas without slipping.

Encourage your partner to close his or her eyes, so as to focus on your touch. Also, it can be disconcerting to have someone staring up at you, especially as a novice.

1. Begin by stroking up each side of the jawline to the forehead. Repeat four or five times.
2. Slowly stroke the forehead rhythmically with the flat of your hand from just above the brows to the hairline.
3. Starting at the centre hairline slide your thumbs out to the side, applying gentle pressure. Move down the forehead slightly and repeat. Continue this outward stroking pressure until you reach the eyebrows.
4. Now place the heel of each hand on the centre forehead and slide out to the sides. Repeat three times.
5. Place the first two fingers of each hand on the temples and circle gently for a minute or two, applying a little pressure.

All the above movements help to relieve a headache. Try lavender oil for your massage, as I've found it can ward off a headache if used in time.

6. Place your thumbs on your partner's inner eyebrows and slide out to the sides. Repeat three times.
7. With your index finger and thumb gently pull along the brow bone. Repeat three times.
8. Stroke gently over the eyelids with your ring fingers, from the inner to the outer corners. Repeat three times.
9. Alternately stroke down the nose with your thumbs, then gently rub round the nose tip and nostrils. Be careful not to press hard on the nostrils.
10. Stroke the cheeks across the cheekbones and gradually work down the face to the chin.
11. Make little circular movements across the top lip. When you reach the corner of the mouth lift slightly, then repeat.
12. Make pinching movements out along the jawline and up towards the ears.
13. Rub the earlobes between your fingers and thumb, then gently pinch all around the outer ear. Most people love this.
14. Sweep your hands up the neck and on to the cheeks. Hold, then repeat.
15. Finish by stroking the forehead, getting lighter and lighter until you bring your hands off.

Scalp Movements

1. Remove your partner's headband. Bring your hands up the side of the face to the forehead, then rake them through the hair. Repeat several times.

2. 'Glue' your fingers onto the scalp and move it around against the skull. Move your fingers to a different position and repeat this process until all the scalp has been covered.
3. Rub vigorously over the scalp, as if shampooing the hair.
4. Take little bunches of hair all over the scalp and tug gently. This feels lovely and really stimulates the scalp.
5. Repeat step 1 to finish off.

• • •

27

Yogic Kriyas to Detoxify the Body and Relieve Pain

These Yogic Kriyas are the purification processes of the body by yogic methods. They are very important in Yoga. Union of body with mind, union of mind with soul and union of soul with God is Yoga.

Kriyas are to be practised early in the morning before rise on empty stomach. Kriyas must be finished before starting the Asanas or Pranayama.

Among these kriyas only Kapalbhati is not related to water. All other five kriyas are water related and helpful in eliminating several disorders.

These Kriyas consist of six purification practises -

1. Dhauti (Kunjal)
2. Basti
3. Neti
4. Tratak
5. Nauli, and
6. Kapalbhati.

Dhauti (Kunjal)

Vomit-Dhauti-Cleaning. Washing stomach by water.

Two or three litre of tepid water is required. Squat on your feet back, spine and neck should be straight. Drink glasses of tepid water continuously without any pause upto the brim of neck. One should neither talk nor laugh during this period. He should not bend and should stand.

Bend a bit forward. Keep the left hand on the left knee and the first and second finger of the right hand in your throat. Press the stomach by the other hand. You will vomit. Vomit the whole drunk water. Water should not remain in stomach.

Wash your hands and take rest. Milk or breakfast should be taken after an hour.

This Dhauti kriya should be practised after passing stool and after bath. One should not take bath after this kriya. Vaman Dhauti kriya should be practised once a fortnight or once a month.

Precautions - 1. Heart patients should not practise it. 2. The nails of the fingers should be trimmed otherwise they may wound the throat.

Benefits - 1. Disorders of bile and gas are cured. 2. It is beneficial in the diseases of stomach throat and jaundice.

BASTI (ENEMA)

Enema pot, rubber tube, nozzle, tepid water, lemon are the requirements. Mix juice of one or two lemons in the tepid water. Fill the enema pot with water.

Suspend the enema pot one metre above. Apply a little oil or vaseline to the nozzle of the rectal tube. Before insertion, check the rectal tube to ensure free flow of water. Insert the tube into the rectum. The flow of water can be adjusted with the knob attached to the tube. When all the water has been introduced, remove the tube and resist the pressure for a few minutes. The bowels can be emptied after a while for better cleansing. If one does not wish to take enema in the lying position he can take it in the standing position.

Special note - Enema should be taken after going to latrine. Salt can be mixed in water instead of lemon juice. You can use plain water also. Soap should not be mixed in water.

Precautions

1. Enema should be taken once in a week or in a month by a healthy person.
2. It can be taken for two to four days daily in constipation.
3. Take rest for half an hour after enema.
4. Do not take any thing after enema for an hour.

Benefits

1. Removes constipation.
2. Cleans bowels.
3. Beneficial in all diseases of stomach.

Neti

It is mainly of two types:

i. Jala Neti ii. Sutra Neti.

Jala Neti

For doing this, squat on your feet. Take tepid salted water in a medium sized pot alongwith spout, made especially for this purpose.

Now fill the pot with tepid salted water and hold it in your right hand to the level of your nose. Then tilt your head slightly to the left so as to have the slanting position of the left nostril. Insert the nozzle of the spout into the right nostril and allow the water to flow down slowly. The water should continue falling down from other nostril in a continuous thin stream. Now repeat the process from the other side. Breath through the mouth only till the kriya is complete. After Jal Neti, stand erect with your feet together. Keep the hands behind your back clasped and blow out vigorously whatever trace of water that has remained in your nostrils.

Precautions - If sometimes one feels intolerable pain in the back of ear or above nostrils, he should practise the Kriya of Kapalbhati at once. It will cure the pain.

Water can come out of eyes in beginning of Neti. These can be warmed. Do not fear.

Benefits

- It cures sinusitis and clears sinuses.
- It cures diseases of nose, eyes, throat and prevents the occurrence of diseases.
- It purifies mind.
- It improves memory.
- It cures coryza and removes old accumulated phlegm.

Sutra Neti or Rubber Neti

Sutra Neti is performed with a 12 inches long piece of waxed cord. It is partly twisted and it makes the nasal insertion possible.

Squat on your feet. Take tepid salted water and soak the Neti well in it. Now take the waxed and twisted end of the cord and make it to curve. Bend your head slightly forward and insert the end of the cord into the nostril through which you have been breathing at that time. Push the cord gradually through the nose, down the throat. Now open your mouth wide, put your index and middle fingers in and with their tips catch the inside end of the cord and draw it out. Hold both the ends in your hand separately and pull the cord very gently up and down three to four times. Then take it out, wash it and then repeat the cycle with the other nostril.

After completion of the kriya, wash the cord with soap well and leave it to dry in some clean and safe place so that the flies, etc. do not pollute it.

Special note

- When the cord reaches throat through nostrils, it becomes greasy by mucus. Therefore, both the ends of the cord should be caught firmly.
- Sutra Neti or Rubber Neti should be practised after learning Jal Neti. After this one can practise Neti with milk, oil or ghee.
- It is more beneficial to perform this Sutra Neti by cotton cord but it should be wrapped.

Precautions

- One can sneeze in practising Sutra Neti. Water can come out of eyes. One should not fear. Practice makes one perfect.
- Nose can bleed sometimes while performing Sutra Neti. In such conditions use rubber catheter (No. 4) instead of cotton cord. Move the cord through nostrils and throat slowly and gently.

Benefits

- It cures all diseases of nose.
- It reduces polyp in nose.
- It cures sinusitis.
- It cures coryza.
- It improves eyesight.
- It improves memory.
- It purifies mind.

Nasapan

Drinking water through nostrils is called nasapan. One should clean the nostrils before drinking water through them.

Milk Neti

Milk is used in place of water. Milk should be without malai cream.

Benefits - Nasapan prevents cold and coryza. It improves eyesight.

Oil Neti

Mustard oil should be made warm in a spoon. When it is lukewarm and tolerable to the skin, lie down on a bed and drip five or seven drops of oil through some dropper in both the nostrils and try to draw them in. You will feel that the oil going in. You can use clean cotton instead of dropper. Coconut or almond oil can be used in place of mustard oil. Pure ghee can also be used. Three or four drops of ghee or Badam Rogan are sufficient for the nostrils.

Oil Neti or Neti of ghee should be done before going to bed at night.

Benefits - It lubricates noses and cleanses it. It prevents from cold and coryza.

Tratak

It is an amazing exercise to improve your power of concentration and eyesight.

It can be practised with a candle or with a black dot on a piece of paper fixed on the wall. Start this practice in a closed room, as there will be less objects to disturb your concentration.

Sit on floor in any comfortable of Padmasana pose. Keep your back and spinal cord erect. Have a few deep breaths. Make your breath steady, even and rhythmic. Keep the object of your gaze at your eye level at a distance of three to four feet. Keep the eyes meditatively wide out of your eyes. Close the eyes to let tears trickle down.

Now mentally visualize that object when the mental image visualizes, open your eyes and start gazing afresh. Do not strain your nerves and get relaxed. Let not your mind wander. Try to bring your mind back to the object but without straining yourself much as that would sap your energy and you will be tired soon.

After practising with the point on the walls or on a steady flame, try to-do it concentrating on the tip of your nose on the point between the eyebrows.

Benefits

1. Tartar improves eyesight and removes the diseases of eyes.
2. It helps in concentrating your mind.
3. It purifies your mind.

Nauli Kriya

It is the best exercise for preserving and promoting the health of abdominal viscera.

- Nauli is equal to Uddiyana Bandh.
- Nauli should be practised daily in the morning on empty stomach and evacuated bowels.
- Stand with legs one foot apart. Bend the legs a little and stoop forward. Rest the palms on thighs just above your knees, with fingers spread. Press the thighs well with your palms and the chest with your chin at the notch between the collar bones.

- Inhale deeply and exhale vigorously so as to force out all the air from the lungs.
- Suspend the breath and pull the abdominal region back towards the spine so that a hollow is formed.
- Push the abdominal recti forward so that a vertical ridge down the centre is formed. Remain in this position for a few seconds and then relax the gap and inhale smoothly.
- Breath deeply three to four times and then repeat the cycle. Repeat it five to seven times.

Special Note

1. Nauli kriya is not easy. Obese persons feel difficulty in its practise. It is essential to practice Uddiyana Bandh and Agnisar to perform Nauli.
2. Nauli kriya should be performed on empty stomach after cleaning bowels and before taking food.
3. One should wear only underwear while practising Nauli. Women can wear bra/ brassiere also.

Precautions

1. Nauli should be practised on empty stomach.
2. It should not be practised unless there is some expert to demonstrate and then to guide and supervise the whole process.
3. It should not be practised before the age of 12 or 13 years.
4. The ulcer patient and the weak person should perform Nauli on the advice of Yoga therapist.
5. The patients suffering from swelling of intestines, dysentery, hernia and high blood pressure should not practice Nauli.

Benefits - The benefits of Nauli are many. It strengthens the abdominal muscles and liver. Women who suffer from a menstrual problem get immediate relief. It increases gastric fire and helps eliminating the toxic elements from the digestive system. It also helps in ovarian insufficiency. Nauli quickly cures constipation, dyspepsia, flatulence etc.

KAPALBHATI

Kapal means skull. Bhati means shine or lustre. Thus, this term means "skull shining". Kapalbhati is a Pranayama also besides one of the six cleaning exercises. Actually this kriya or cleansing process is a milder form of Bhastrika, another vigorously breathing exercise.

Sit on a blanket or a dari in Padmasana, Sidhasana or Sukhasana. Keep back, spinal cord and neck erect. Keep both the hands on knees. Shut your eyes. Sit peacefully. Exhale vigorously. Do not inhale. At start begin slowly after four to five exhales. Exhale vigorously and quickly. Be careful in exhaling; you will inhale between exhales.

One should not pause during the practice of Kapalbhati. Hold the breath after exhaling (Kumbhak). During Kumbhak practice Jallandhar Bandh, Uddiyana Bandh, Mool Bandh and Mahabandh. Hold this position for a while. Release all Bandhs and inhale slowly. This completes one round of Kapalbhati. Start with two rounds. You can practice unto five rounds gradually. Start with ten or twelve exhales. Gradually you can increase their number 50 to 120.

SPECIAL NOTE-

1. The stomach should go inside at once after exhaling.
2. The difference between Kapalbhati and Bhasrika Pranayam is that both inhale and exhale are done vigorously. One should learn it from an expert in Yogic Kriya.

Precautions - Persons with high BP problems or pus in the ear should refrain from doing this exercise.

Benefits - This Kapalbhati is very good invigorating exercise which cleanses the entire respiratory system by forcefully rushing exhalation.

It removes concentration and mental retention. The movement of the diaphragm stimulates the stomach, heart liver and spleen. This exercise is very good for eyes.

Agnisar

The practice of Agnisar kindles energy in stomach and body perspires.

Sit on a blanket or dari in Vajrasana. Keep a little distance between the knees. Put firmly both the hands on the knees. Inhale vigorously and while exhaling shrink your stomach as much as you can. Now suspend your breath. It is called Bahya Kumbhak.

Holding the position of Bahya Kumbhak, i.e. keeping the breath suspended and pulling the entire abdominal region back towards your spine. Now blow your stomach out and shrink in. In one Kumbhak you can blow and shrink your stomach 8-20 times .

This kriya is called Agnisar. One can practice this kriya in a standing posture.

Benefits -

1. Cures obesity.
2. Cures disorders of abdominal region.
3. It improves lack of appetite.

Bandh

Bandh means binding. Bandhs literally means a lock, bondage or joining together to objects or stages. A Bandh is a special posture invented to conserve and make greater use of vast resources of energy generated by yogic exercises and Pranayama. These Bandhs are means of reorientation and control of the vital energy of your body and mind. These are of three main types.

Jalandhar Bandh

In this Bandh the throat is contracted blocked, as it were, by making the chin rest on the chest in the notch between the collar bones in certain asanas or posture like Sarvangasana exhalation and fresh, when the breath is suspended. Once in a day early in the morning it should be practised, first standing, then in advanced stage in the sitting position.

Stand erect with your feet one foot apart. Bend the knees a little and then slightly bend forward. Rest your palms with fingers spread on your thigh above the knees. Take a few deep breaths and then exhale forcefully. This is automatically practised. In these postures the chin is firmly pressed against the chest. This chin lock regulates the flow of blood to the heart, head, brain and neck. Jalandhar Bandh is also practised in combination with Mula Bandh.

Uddiyana Bandh

It is a very powerful Bandh and a basic for regulating the flow of prana and awakening of Kundalini. Uddiyana involves the lifting of the diaphragm high up the chest and pulling up the abdominal organs towards the spine. It means to fly up. This Bandh makes the great bird of Prana fly towards the highest chakra Brahmarandhara or Sahasara. Inhale upto fill and exhale so as to empty your lungs completely.

Keep the breath suspended and pull the entire abdominal region back towards your spine. Then draw it up toward thorax. Keep the pressure of your palms on the thighs all this time. Remain in the pose for 20-30 seconds according to your capacity.

Relax the grip on your abdominal region and inhale slowly and deeply. Repeat the cycle three to five times.

Benefits

- Uddiyana Bandh is of great spiritual value as it forces the Prana upto Sushumna nadi.
- It invigorates the whole abdominal region.
- It is said to rejuvenate an old person, if it is properly and constantly practised.
- The uplifting of diaphragm massages the heart muscles.

Mula Bandh

Mula literally means the root, source, foundation or the basis. In it the portion between anus and scrotum is contracted and raised. This prevents Apana escaping from the lower body and draws it up to unite with Prana.

Sit in Padmasana or Sidhasan. Stretch your hands and fingers as if in Gyan mudra. Now inhale deeply and retain your breath. Press the chin against the chest in the chin lock. Now contract the region of lower abdomen between the anus and the navel towards your spine and pull it upwards towards the diaphragm. The contract and pull towards the abdominal muscles and remain in the posture for a few seconds. Now release the grip on abdominal muscles and remove the chin lock. Exhale slowly and evenly. Repeat the cycle three to five times.

Benefits

- It cures piles.
- It cures the disorders of intestines
- It prevents Apana vayu (foul wind) escaping from the lower body and raw it to unite with the Prana vayu (the vital wind).

- It increases sexual retention power which we sublimated makes a man 'Urdhuvaretus'
- It also helps in awakening the dormant Kundalini.

The Mula Bandh should be practised when one becomes perfect in doing certain difficult asanas like Sirshansa, Sarvasana etc.

Maha Bandh

Sit in Padmasana on a blanket. Shut your eyes. Now practise Jalandhar, Uddiyaana and Mula Bandh together.

Benefits

- You get the benefit of all the three Bandhs at once by Maha Bandh.
- It cures the menstrual problems of ladies.
- It cures ovarian problems of ladies.
- It helps in strength mixing sex organs of males.

• • •

28

Dietary and Juice Cure of Osteoarthritis, Rheumatoid Arthritis, Backache

Osteoarthritis

Osteoarthritis is a form of arthritis affecting the bones and joints. It is characterized by mild early-morning stiffness, stiffness after periods of rest, pain that is worse when the joint is used and loss of joint function. Symptoms can range from local tenderness, swelling of soft tissues, bony swelling and restricted mobility to cracking of joints in movement. Osteoarthritis is divided into two categories-primary and secondary. Primary osteoarthritis is a degenerative condition brought about by wear and tear on the body. Secondary osteoarthritis is brought about by predisposing factors such as trauma or previous inflammatory disease of the joint.

General Recommendations

Osteoarthritis sufferers should achieve and maintain normal body weight. Excess weight places an added strain on the weight-bearing joints. For some individuals, symptoms disappear completely after weight loss.

Dietary Modifications

- Try eliminating the nightshade family-tomatoes, peppers, potatoes, eggplant and tobacco. If symptoms improve even slightly, continue to avoid these foods. Though not proven, there is a theory that a long-term low-level consumption of the solanum, alkaloids found in this family inhibits normal collagen repair in the joints or encourages inflammatory degeneration of the joints,

- Avoid the citrus family-lemons, limes, oranges and grapefruits. This family, like the nightshade family, is thought to contribute to joint swelling.
- Avoid all refined foods such as white flour, white sugar and preserved and processed foods. Eat a nutritious diet that emphasizes whole grains, legumes (beans, split peas and lentils), seeds, nuts, vegetables, and fruits includes only a small portion of low-fat animal products.
- Significantly decrease your consumption of sweets and alcohol.
- Consider testing for food allergies.
- Check for hydrochloric acid deficiency. Seek medical advice in this regard.
- Try a juice fast, which has been shown to be very helpful for arthritis.

Nutrients That Help

- Niacinamide may bring a noticeable improvement within two to six weeks. This nutrient is said to be especially beneficial for degenerative arthritis of the knee. (Waming, Niacinamide supplements may affect the liver or cause nausea.)
- Pantothenic acid may be helpful, as a deficiency of this nutrient has been associated with osteoarthritis.
- Vitamin C may be beneficial.
- Vitamin E may produce effects similar to those of nonsteroidal anti-inflammatory drugs.
- Methionine is important in cartilage structures.

- Superoxide dismutase may have therapeutic benefits.
- Copper may be helpful, as a deficiency of this nutrient has been associated with osteoa.
- Bioilavonolds have been shown to be beneficial.
- Bromelain has anti-inflammatory properties.

Beneficial Juices

- Broccoli and kale-sources of pantothenic acid.
- Kale, parsley and spinach-sources of vitamin C.
- Spinach and carrot-sources of vitamin E.
- Carrot, ginger root and apple-sources of copper.
- Cherry and blueberry-sources of bioflavonoids.
- Pineapple--the only source of bromelain.

Suggested Juicing Recipes for Osteoarthritis

Digestive Special

Handful spinach
4-5 carrots, greens removed

Bunch up spinach and push through hopper with carrots

Broccoli - Garlic Special

3 broccoli flowerets
1 garlic clove
4-5 carrots or 2 tomatoes
2 stalks celery
½ green pepper

Push broccoli and garlic through hopper with carrots or tomatoes. Follow with celery and green pepper.

Blueberry - Grape Special

1 quart blueberries
1 medium bunch grapes
1/4-inch slice ginger root

Push blueberries through hopper, followed by grapes and ginger. Pour juice into

Sparkling water	ice-filled glass. Fill glass to top with sparkling water.

Pineapple - Ginger Special

1/4 pineapple with skin	Push pirte apple
Ginger Hopper	through hopper.
1/4-inch slice ginger root	Push ginger through hopper
4-5 carrots, greens removed	with carrots and apple.
1/2 apple, seeded	

Rheumatoid Arthritis

Rheumatoid arthritis is a systemic disease characterized by inflammatory changes in joints and related structures. Its symptoms include fatigue, low-grade fever, weakness joint stiffness and pain. There is often severe joint pain, with increased inflammation beginning in small joints and progressively affecting all joints in the body. Evidence exists that rheumatoid arthritis is an auto immune reaction in which antibodies develop against components of joint tissues.

Dietary Modifications

- Consume a low-fat, low-calorie diet excluding most animal sources (meat, dairy products and so forth). Studies have shown that patients following this type of diet experienced remission of joint symptoms. A vegetarian diet, excluding all animal sources but fish, has been found to be very beneficial.
- Increase your consumption of cold-water fish, e.g., mackerel, salmon tuna, and sardines. Cod-liver oil may also be beneficial.
- Exclude refined sugar, refined wheat flour, cornflour, salt, strong spices, alcohol, tea and coffee from your diet.

- Identify food allergies.
- Check for low stomach acid (hydrochloric acid). See your doctor for testing.
- One folk remedy calls for drinking basil as a tea. Basil has been used to ease rheumatoid pain.
- Try a Juice fast, which has been shown to help arthritis.

Nutrients That Help

- Vitamin C has anti-inflammatory action.
- Vitamin- E has anti-inflammatory action.
- Vitamins may stabilize the membranes and cells of rheumatoid tissue.
- Pantothenic acid may be helpful, as deficiencies of this nutrient have been found to be directly related to symptoms.
- Copper has anti-inflammatory action.
- Iron may be helpful, as an iron deficiency may be involved. (Supplementation is controversial. Food is the best source.)
- Manganese may have therapeutic benefits.
- Selenium may be helpful, as a deficiency may be involved.
- Sulphur may be helpful, as a deficiency may be involved.
- Zinc may be helpful, as a deficiency may be involved.
- Bromelain has anti-inflammatory properties.
- Omega-3 fatty acids have therapeutic benefits.
- Superoxide dismutase has anti-inflammatory properties.

Beneficial Juices

- Parsley, broccoli. and spinach-sources of vitamin C.
- Spinach, carrot, and tomato-sources of vitamin E.

- Broccoli, lettuce, and cabbage-sources of vitamin K.
- Broccoli and kale-sources of pantothenic acid.
- Carrot, ginger root and apple-sources of copper.
- Parsley, beet greens and broccoli-sources of iron.
- Spinach, beet greens, carrot, turnip, orange and grape-sources of manganese.
- Ginger root, parsley and carrot-sources of selenium.
- Cabbage and kale-sources of sulphur.
- Ginger root, parsley, garlic and carrot-sources of zinc.
- Pineapple-the only source of bromelain.
- Dark green vegetables-sources of omega-3 fatty acids.

Suggested Juicing Recipes For Rheumatoid Arthritis

SPINACH - CARROT SPECIAL

Small handful spinach	Bunch up spinach and push
4-5 carrots, greens removed	through hopper with carrots
½ apple, seed	and apple.

GARDEN SALAD SPECIAL

3 broccoli flowerets	Push broccoli and garlic
1 garlic clove	through hopper with carrots
4-5 carrots or 2 tomatoes	or tomatoes. Follow with
2 stalks celery	celery and green pepper
Bromelain green pepper	

GINGER-CARROT SPECIAL

1/4-inch slice ginger root	Push ginger through hopper
4-5 carrots, greens removed	with carrots and apple.
¼ apple seeded	

Pineapple special

1/4 pineapple, with skin
½ apple, seeded
1/4-inch slice ginger root

Push pineapple through hopper with apple and ginger.

Ginger Berry Special

1 quart blueberries
1 medium bunch grapes
Winch slice ginger root
Sparkling water

Push blueberries through hopper, followed by grapes and ginger. Pour juice into ice filled glass.

Potassium Broth

Handful parsley
Handful spinach
4-5 carrots, greens
removed 2 stalks celery

Bunch up parsley and spinach leaves, and push through hopper with carrots and celery.

Cleansing Cocktail

1/4-inch slice ginger root
1 beet
¼ apple, seeded
4 carrots greens removed

Push ginger, beet and apple through hopper with carrots.

Backache

Backache is a common syndrome characterized by pain and tenderness in the muscles or in the muscles' attachments to other regions, such as the sacroiliac. Back pain is a signal that something is wrong in the body. It can be caused by infection, disorders of the vertebral column, or a number of other conditions, -including stress. Back pain is a sign to take action and seek professional medical advice. There are some things you can do in addition to help the healing process.

GENERAL RECOMMENDATIONS

From a psychological standpoint, much can be done to help control back pain. For example, focusing, relaxation methods and biofeed back can all be very helpful. In addition, physical therapy, massage and acupuncture have provided therapeutic benefits. Diet may not have much influence on how one perceives back pain, but it can be very important in the healing process. An exception would be certain herbal remedies that have been used throughout history in the treatment of pain, such as red pepper, clove oil, German chamomile, and wintergreen oil. Traditionally, chestnuts also have been used to relieve backache.

DIETARY MODIFICATIONS

- Reduce your consumption of animal fats. In decreasing your consumption of these fats, you will decrease your intake of arachidonic acid, which contributes to the inflammatory process.
- Eat more fatty cold-waterfish, such as mackerel, herring, and salmon. These fish contain a substance that has anti-inflammatory properties.
- Avoid instant coffee. A study has shown that instant coffee blocks certain receptor sites in the brain that naturally help the body control pain. When these receptor sites are blocked, the body is more susceptible to pain.
- Follow one of the cleansing diets. Many people have experienced pain relief and healing from injuries during and after a cleansing diet. Cherie experienced a great deal

of pain after a car accident in which she sustained whiplash injuries. After six months of therapy without much improvement, she went on a three-day juice fast, after which her condition greatly improved.

Nutrients that Help

- Vitamin K has shown some promising results in pain management in studies not yet published.
- Copper deficiency can contribute to pain perception.
- D-phenylalaniwi, an amino acid, may effectively ease chronic pain even when medications offer no relief. Speak to your doctor about supplementation.

Beneficial Juices

- Turnip greens, broccoli, lettuce, cabbage and spinach - sources of vitamin K.
- Carrot, garlic, and ginger root-sources of copper.

Suggested Juicing Recipes for Backache

Vegetables - Apple Special

2 lettuce leaves	Bunch up lettuce leaves and
1 small wedge cabbage	push through hopper with
4-5 carrots, greens removed	cabbage, carrots, broccoli,
3 broccoli flowerets	and apple.
½ apple, seeded	

Ginger Carrot Special

¼ inch slice ginger root	Push ginger through hopper
4-5 carrots, greens removed	with carrots and apple.
½ apple, seeded	

Ginger Apple Special

1/4-inch slice ginger root 1 apple, seeded Sparkling water	Push ginger through hopper with apple. Pour-juice into ice-filled glass. Fill, glass to top with sparkling water.

Potassium Special

Handful parsley Handful spinach 4-5 carrots, greens removed 2 stalks celery	Bunch up parsley and spinach leaves, and push through hopper with carrots and celery.

Digestive Special

Handful spinach 4-5 carrots, greens removed	Bunch up spinach and push through hopper with carrots.

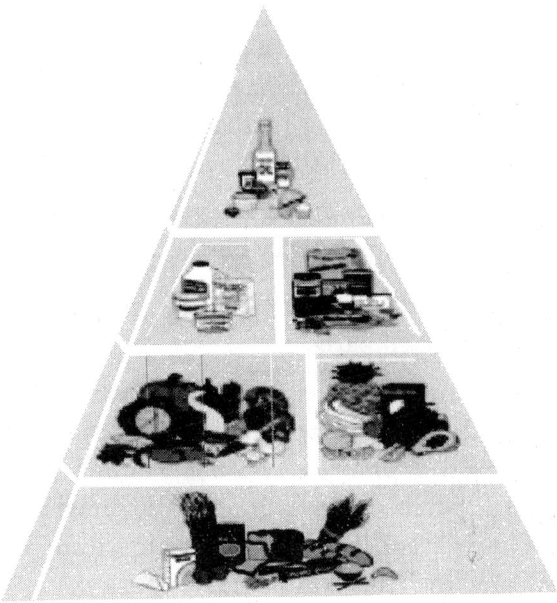

29

Ayurvedic Treatment for Pain of Muscles and Joints

In our daily life, we suffer from sprain, backache and body aches. Here are the remedies for various muscular & joint disorders:-

Muscular Cramps

- Apply clove oil on the affected parts.

Sprain

- Chop raw onions and put in a towel. Place this over the sprain to relieve pain and bring down the swelling. Alternatively, make a footbath of lavender oil and water and soak your ankle, but do not massage the area.
- Grind lime leaves into a fine paste. Mix it with an equal quantity of butter. Apply on the affected areas.
- Mix equal parts of almonds oil & garlic oil and massage over the affected parts.
- Take 1 gram flour, just a pinchful, and add half of its quantity with equal amount of turmeric powder. Add linseed oil in it or any other oil like of mustard or til, and make the poultice . Apply it on the sprained portion. The poultice will enhance the blood circulation and in two days' time the relief will be there.

Muscular Pain

- Warm the papaya leaf over the fire and apply on affected parts.
- Heat ginger (adrak) paste with turmeric (haldi) paste (1:1) and apply.
- Soak ½ teaspoon liquoric (mulathi) root powder in 1 cup water and leave overnight. Mix into the infusion 1 cup rice gruel (cooked broken rice) and take every morning.

Rib Pain

- Grind a turmeric piece and mix in a hot water to form a thick paste. Apply this paste over the ribs aching. Soon the pain will vanish. In case you feel you are not having the desired effect, prepare the oil of turmeric and lightly massage your aching ribs with this oil. Another treatment for quick relief is to mix turmeric powder in the milk of the Aak plant (the medicinal plant, swallow wort, whose botanical name is Calotropes Gigantea) and apply over the ribs. This paste will quickly give relief.

Ankle Swelling & Pain

- Mix equal quantities of castor oil and lime juice. Massage the affected area with the mixture. Also drink 1 cup warm water mixed with lime juice and honey.

Heels having Pain

- Mix equal amounts by weight of carom seeds (ajwain) onion seeds (kalaunji), fenugreek seeds (methi daana) and saboot isabgol. Have 1 tablespoon everyday first thing in the morning. If you can grind them slightly in the mixer - makes it more effective. This treatment takes a couple of months but is a sure shot remedy.

Note: Saboot isabgol, tiny very light pinkish particles, will be available with your grocer or if you request him he will get it for you from the wholesale market. Do not use the husk which is generally used by people for constipation as that is less effective but not harmful. If saboot isabgol is not available, husk can be used. It takes longer for the pain to go.

Legs, Swelling and Pain

- Mix equal quantities of castor oil and lime juice. Massage the affected area with this mixture. Also drink 1 cup warm water mixed with lime juice and honey.

Athletes's Foot

Keeping your feet clean and dry is enough to discourage the growth of this fungal infection. Remember, it is infectious and you must keep and wash your shoes, socks, and towel separately. To sooth the broken areas of your feet, simply soak them for 10 minutes in a foot-both of apple cider vinegar mixed with water.

Foot Corns

- Tie a fresh slice of lemon over the corn (painful area) and keep it all night.
- Massage castor oil on the corns every morning and night before sleeping.
- Massage for 2-3 minutes so that the oil gets absorbed. In 3-4 weeks the corns will disappear.
- Mash 1-2 cloves (laung) & garlic (lahasun) and tie over the corns. Keep overnight.

Sciatica

- Take just 10 gms. of turmeric and grind it in 100 gms. of cow's urine. Add about 25 gms. of castor oil to it and make the patient drink the whole lot. The patient will get relief. Alternatively make the patient inhale deeply the vapours emerging out of the large vessel in which jaggery is being prepared from the sugar cane juice. But the patient must keep his body covered with a heavy blanket. The more he sweats, the quicker he will be cured.

Paralysis

- Boil a few leaves of tulsi in a tumbler full of water. When cool, strain and put this water in a bottle. Massage this water on the affected limbs. Continue this treatment for at least two weeks. This treatment, coupled with regular intake of the tulsi leaves as an alternative treatment along with other remedies is helpful in giving good results.

Fainting

- A hot poultice of carom seeds (ajwain) may be used as dry fomentation for hands and feet.

Fatigue

- Take a glass of grapefruit and lemon juice in equal parts to dispel fatigue and general tiredness after a days' work.

Body Weakness

- Soak 8 to 10 almonds and 1 teaspoon rice overnight. Remove the outer skin of almonds. Grind into a fine paste. Mix in some milk and pinch of turmeric powder (haldi) . Boil and drink along with sugar candy (mishri) or ordinary sugar to taste.
- Sprinkle the following on a platter of mango slices; 1 teaspoon honey, a pinch of saffron (kesar), cardamom (chhoti illaichi) and rose water (gulab jal). Take twice daily.

Exhaustion Due to Overwork

- Boil ¼ teaspoon powdered cardamom (chhoti illaichi) seeds in thin tea water and drink.

Gout-Swelling

- Take 250 gms. of turmeric powder, 50 gms; Kuchala powder, 50gms; pigeon dung, 100 gms; castor oil and 250gms. til oil. Mix both the oils, add turmeric, kuchala and pigeons dung and boil. When the solid contents turn black, cool and strain the oil mixture. Add to it a cup of kerosene oil. Repeatedly massage this oil on your joints. Always massage the adjoining areas before massaging the swollen part. Like if you have to massage your knees, first massage the upper thigh and thigh joint before massaging the knees. This way the raw phlegm will be dissolved and not shifted to other portion. Try not to have constipation when you take this massage course.

Gouty Pains

- Mix mustard oil and rectified alcohol (1 part oil to 40 parts alcohol) and use as a lotion.
- Make a poultice of ground fenugreek seeds (methi dana) use on the affected part.
- Equal quantities of Asparagus seeds (halong). Black cumin, fenugreek (methi) and Ajwain should be taken and swallowed every morning in dose of 3 grams. The remedies are also recommended for rheumatism and lumbago.

Rheumatism

- Heat the leaves of the plant swallow wort (Aak in Hindi) and tie them over the affected joints.

- Grind the guava leaves to a paste form and apply on the affected joint.
- Take about 750 gms. of the root of Arand plant and boil it in 6kgs. of water. When it is reduced to 1/4th of its normal quantity, then add castor oil to it and boil again till whole of the water in the mixture evaporates leaving only the oily substance. Strain this oil through a fine muslin cloth and keep it preserved, in a glass bottle. Massage your limbs with this oil at least 15mts. before you go to have your bath. In case you do it after your bath, then tie cotton wads after the massage over the affected joints.
- Take 'Binaules', cut, grind and sieve them and boil in water, when only thick paste remains. Dry it and then tie it over your affected joints.

Rheumatic Pain

- Boil 3 tablespoon powdered nutmeg (jaiphal) in 1 cup sesame oil (til ka tel). Cool and apply on affected parts.
- 2 to 3 teaspoon pepper powder is fried in 2 teaspoons sesame oil (til ka tel) until charred. When it is warm, it is applied on the affected areas and massaged lightly.
- A 3 inch piece of dried ginger is grinded with a grape sized piece of asafoetida (hing) in milk. The paste is applied on the affected area. The area is exposed to the sun for imparting warmth and heat.
- The patient must avoid fried eatables and sour foods like curds and alcohol, moong dal, meat soup, garlic, onions, bitter gourd, papaya and green bananas are the foods which help in controlling gout and rheumatic pain.

Joint Pain

- Take equal quantities of asparagus seeds (shatavari), black cumin seeds (shah jeera), fenugreek (methi daana) seeds and carom seeds (ajwain). Powder and take 1/2 teaspoon every morning.
- Combine 6 teaspoons each of ginger (adrak) and caraway seeds along with 3 teaspoons of black pepper corns (saboot kali mirch) and grind into a fine powder. Have ½ teaspoon with water twice daily.
- Soak 1-2 teaspoons fenugreek seeds (methi daana) in a cup of curd overnight. Eat in the morning on an empty stomach or soak 1-2 teaspoons fenugreek seeds (methi daana) in 1 cup water overnight. Drink the water first thing in the morning and also eat the methi seeds.
- Take out 1 tablespoon juice of fresh leaves of bathua and drink every day on an empty stomach for 2-3 months. Do not add anything to the juice and do not eat anything before and after, for 2 hours.
- Make a tea from papaya seeds and have 6-7 cups a day, for at least 2 weeks.
- Have 1-2 garlic (lahasun) cloves or 1 garlic, which has only 1 clove in a pod, first thing in the morning.
- Mix 1 teaspoon of dry amla powder with 2 teaspoons of jaggery (gur) and have it twice daily for a month.

Arthritis

Extract the juice of carrots and add to it the juice of Karnphool (Dandelion). Have just 5 gms. of carrot juice and add only half of the quantity the juice of dandelion. Drink this combination regularly for at least 15 days for speedier relief. It is also advisable to rub Mahanarayani oil on the joints.

Bed Sores

- Apply honey on the length and breadth of a banana leave and lie on it for a few hours. Ensure its contact with the affected parts.

Body Pain

- Boil 3 tablespoons powdered nutmeg (jaiphal) in 1 cup sesame oil (til ka tel), cool it and apply on affected parts.

• • •

30

Pain in Joints–Homoeopathic Remedies

Ammon Carb: tearing pain in joints, in ankle, and bones of feet, worse evening, cold, wet weather and heat of bed.

Angustura: tension and stiffness in joints and muscles, worse walking.

Kali-Bich: shifting pain in joints, worse morning and cold.

Kali-Sil: feeling of stiffness and creeping in joints and limbs with desire to lie down, worse cold bath and open air.

Kalm: pain in right shoulder and hip shooting downward with feeling of tingling, numbness and coldness worse motion and open air.

Kreos: pain in joints, often in hips and knees, worse open air and rest.

Lac Can: when pain changes sides of the body.

Lac. ac: pain in joints particularly in shoulders, wrists and knees with copious urine and feeling of weekness.

Euon: pain in joints, more in ankles, worse evening and cool air.

Magnol: shifting pain in joints with feeling of numbness, worse morning, rest and damp-cold.

Paraffin: shifting, knife-like, tearing, wrenching or electric-like shocks in joints, more in ankles and soles, obstinate constipation, pains sometimes in alternation with stomach or heart trouble.

Pinus-s: pain in joints, more in finger joints with stiffness and cramps in calves, itching about joints.

Radium: severe pain in joints and limbs worse night, better by hot bath, open air, walking, pressure.

Form-r: pain in joints more on hips with stiffness and feeling of contraction, worse by cold damp; better after midnight, rubbing.

Phos-ac: pain in joints and bones, loss of vital fluids - **China** worse night, better by warmth.

Aur-Met: tearing pain in joints with profound despondency and disgust of life, worse cold and night.

Bar-c: pain in joints in old age, blood pressure, better in open air

Apoc: pain in joints, soles, toes, cramps, and heat in soles, tingling in toes.

Particular Group of Joints and Limbs Affected

Piper: pain in the thumb joint, right arm, paralytic weakness in hand, worse thinking of it-Ox.ac.

Lil.t: pain in hip, ankle, right arm, legs better in open air.

Sol-lye: pain in right shoulder, arm: elbow, wrist and lumber region with tingling: worse jar, open air, motion better warm room.

Guaic: pain in shoulders, arms and hands, worse motion, heat, cold, wet, better by pressure.

Arg-m: pain in knee and elbow with copious urine, better in open air.

Elat: pain in knees, toes, fingers and thumbs worse cold damp.

Hippom: weakness in knees and small joints.

Kali-c: pain in hips, nates and thighs, worse cold, at about 3 a.m.

Note:

1. Gout involves or changes to chest–Colch.
2. Gout involves eyes Nux v., Bell., Rhus-tox., Puls., Acon.
3. Gout involves heart–Aur-m., Cact., Kalm., Colch., Spig., Benz-ac, lith-c., Abrot., Led., Acon., Naja.
4. Gout involves stomach–Hydroc-ac., Nux-m., Nux-v., Puls., Ant. c.
5. Gout involves throat–Colch., Merc-s, Bell., Acon.
6. Gout involves Piles–Abrot.

• • •

31

Single Joints Affected: Homoeopathic Remedies

Abrot: pain in shoulders, worse cold air, rest.

Mag-c: pain in right shoulders, unable to raise arm-Phyt., Sang. c., Rhus-tox., Ferr. met worse rest and cold.

Hyper: pain in shoulders extending downward with tingling, creeping and numbness, worse cold damp.

Inula: pain in right shoulder and wrist with bronchitis and bearing down in female organs.

Phyt: pain in right shoulder, worse night, motion and damp cold.

Spirenth: pain in shoulders with swelling of veins of hands.

Stict-p: pain in right shoulder, with red swelling, worse change of temperature.

Stront-c: pain in right shoulder, worse cold, when begins to move-change of temperature.

Ferr-met: pain in left shoulder, worse at rest better by walking slowly.

Coloc: pain in L shoulder, better by external pressure.

Rhus-tox: pain in shoulders with sleeplessness, worse at rest, damp cold, better during walking.

Asper: pain in left shoulder, radiating downward with cardiac weakness.

Onos: pain in left shoulder with feeling of weakness, worse jar, motion.

Agar: pain in left shoulder and arm, worse damp cold, better slow walking.

Sul: pain in left shoulder with heat in palms and soles, worse night, wet and wash.

Pall: pain in right shoulder and right hip often with ovarian trouble.

Kalm: pain of erratic character with numbness and radiating downward, worse motion, on raising the arm.

Knees

Apis: oedematous swelling with sore skin and stinging pain, worse touch, heat, better uncovering, open air, bath.

Kali-c: swelling with stitching pain, worse cold and at about 3 A.M; backache.

Kali-iod: pain in knees with effusion, worse night and cold wet.

Calc-c: swelling of knees in fatty constitution, with sweats on head and hands, worse cold damp.

Calc-f: pain and swelling of knees with rigidity, worse change of weather, rest, better heat and walking.

Sal. ac: pain and swelling, sweats, worse touch, motion.

Benz-ac: pain and swelling, offensive urine worse on uncovering and open air.

Rhodo: pain and swelling in right knee worse night, morning, cold wet, stormy weather.

Mang. acet: swell, painful and itch, worse motion and cold wet.

Rhus-tox: pain with or without swelling, lumbago, worse at rest, cold damp, better during walking.

Cocc. I: pain and swelling worse when flexed.

Arg. m: pain in knee, elbow with copious urine, better in open air.

Melil: pain and numbness worse motion, damp cold, change of weather.

Nat-c: pain and weakness in knees and ankles, with swelling of hands in the morning.

Coloc: pain in left knee, better by pressure.

Elat: pain in knees, toes, thumbs and fingers, worse cold damp.

Hippom: paralytic weakness.

Phyt: pain shooting, shifting, jerking, electric-like shocks, worse cold damp, night, motion.

Caust: pain with contraction of tendons-Rhodo better warmth and wet weather.

Jac. : pain in right knee with stiff muscles in the morning.

Nat-c: hollow of the knee painful-Caust., Lith-c.

Puls: pain and swelling worse evening, warm room, on letting the affected limb hand down-Vip.

Hips and Loins

Aesc: pain in hips and sacrum worse walking and stooping.

Kali-iod: pain in hips at night.

Staph: pain less in hip-joints, more in back and loins, worse morning before rising.

Nat-s: pain in hip joints often in left side, worse stooping and damp cold.

Guac: pain in hip joints with heavy legs, worse motion.

Hipp. ac: pain in hips, back and things worse right side.

Starm: severe pain in left hip better warmth.

Puls: pain in hip joints and loins worse evening, better motion.

Caust: pain in left hip worse cold, walking better warmth.

Kali-c: pain in right hip to knee, feels as if back and legs should give out, worse cold, at about 3 A.M. better walking.

Card-m: pain in hip joints shooting down to buttocks and things.

Iris: shifting pain in left hip, worse evening and at rest.

Irid: pain in left hip to thigh with weak spine and kidney.

Elat: pain in hips with diarrhoea.

Ginseng: pain in loins with stiffness and heaviness in legs worse night.

Chell: r. sided pain in hips, thighs and heels, better by pressure.

Paraffin: pain in loins and spine, shooting down to inguinal region.

Ruta: pain in loins with weakness in hips and things making one difficult to rise from seat, worse lying down, damp cold.

Rhus-tox: pain in loins with restlessness at night, when begins to move, worse damp cold, better walking.

Berb.-v: pain in loins with urinary complaints, worse motion and standing.

Am-m: lumbago worse sitting.

Colch: lumbago, better rest and pressure.

Lactusa: pain in left loin, worse motion.

Aloes: lumbago alternates with headache and aggravation of piles.

Cobalt: pain in back and sacrum worse sitting, better walking and lying down.

Dios: back-ache worse stooping.

Gnaphal: lumbago with numb feeling, better lying on back.

Ankles

Med: ankles easily turn when waling, sycotic history, time passes slowly, i.e. melancholy mood.

Nat-m: ankles easily turn when walking, liability to take cold, craving for salt, easily tired, worse morning, better open air, cold bath.

Calc-p: ankles turn easily, effective calcium metabolism.

Caust: ankles easily turn when walking, with arthritic, rhematic and paralytic trouble.

Cham: ankles easily turn when walking during dentition period, easily excited to anger.

Mang.acet: ankles easily turn when walking, feels better on lying down painful swell and suppurate.

Nat.ars: the trouble is accompanied by nasal catarrh.

Phos: when patient is hot blooded, desires cool places and cool drinks.

Ruta: after sprains.

Sil: patient chilly with defective nutrition.

Pinus: weak ankles in rachitic children.

Nat-C: ankles easily sprained and dislocated.

Nat-Chl: weak ankles and knees, swelling of hands in the morning.

Eucal: pain and nodular swelling worse night.

Euon: pain in ankle worse evening better pressure.

Guaco: pain in ankle shooting upward-Visc, causing lameness, worse cold damp, movement better pressure.

Prop: pain in ankle with inability to stand.

Stront-C: ankle swollen, and painful, veins of hands enlarged, worse cold, on beginning to move.

Verb: neuralgic pain in left ankle.

Led: ankle swollen and painful better by cold application.

Lith-c: pain in ankle when moving about.

Abrot: swelling, emaciation on lower limbs, pricking pain, increased appetite, worse cold damp.

Arg-m: swelling of ankles in diabetic patients.

Elbows

Arg-m: Oleum. j., Guaco, Visc. Wrists Hippem severe pain in wrist with feeling of weakness in hands and fingers.

Plumb: wrist so weak that unable to lift anything, better rubbing and pressure.

Ruta: pain, stiffness and gouty deposits in wrist, worse cold wet, rest.

Bov: weak wrist with inability to hold anything in hand.

Viol-od: pain in wrist worse cool air.

Act-sp: wrist red and swollen worse on movement.

Caul: pain in wrist in females.

Cobalt: pain in wrist with sexual disturbances.

Abrot: pricking pain, swelling and emaciation, worse cold and damp, night.

Fingers and nails

Am-m: pain, shooting, ulcerative, tearing in tips of fingers often in toes also, worse evening.

Bism: tearing pain in tips of fingers under nails, gastric derangement.

Berb. v: neuralgic pain under finger nails, swelling of finger joints, urinary complaints.

Sec-c: fingers and feet turn bluish, pain in finger tips with tingling and numbness better cold and rubbing.

Sars: burning on sides of fingers and toes ; ulceration around ends of fingers, cutting pain under nails.

Elat: pain in joints of fingers, and thumbs worse by wet and cold.

Calc. f: gouty deposits in finger-joints.

El. ac: joints inflamed, feeling of splinter under nails, nails which crumble, worse warmth.

Ginseng: burning in tips of fingers.

Oleand: swelling, stiffness and burning of fingers, sometimes veins of hands swollen.

Pinus: gouty pain in fingers joints.

Ant-c: pain in finger joints, worse heat and wetting, nails brittle–Graph., Sil.

Am-c: fingers swell when arms hanging down.

Bor: throbbing pain in tip of thumb.

All-c: fingers about nails painful.

Colch: finger tips numb and tingling.

Eug: skin recedes from the nails forming pus.

Nat s: swelling around roots of nails.

Cycl: Cramp-like contraction of right thumb and index finger.

Hep-s: finger joints swollen, and nail of great toe painful on slightest pressure.

Piper-m: pain in thumb joint.

Primula-ver: drawing pain in thumb and toe.

Apis-m: hands and finger tips numb.

Graph: deformity and pain in nails.

Sil: ingrowing of toe-nails.

Psor: psutules about finger nails.

Toes

Am-c: Big toe swollen and painful, worse by cold wet.

Benz-ac: pain or lump or swelling in great toe, offensive urine, better uncovering.

Bor: burning in great toe, balls of toes inflamed, hot urine.

Colch: swelling of great toe with sensitiveness to touch worse motion.

Daph: right toe swollen and painful, pain shoots upto the abdomen and heart, worse cold air.

Elat: gouty pain in great toes-Gnaphal, worse damp cold.

Hyper: pain in toes or fingers, shooting upward with tingling, numbness and burning, worse damp cold.

PIb: pain in right big toe at night, worse touch.

Prim-v: pain in big toe and thumb.

Led: ball of great toe swollen with throbbing worse by heat.

Rhodo: pain and gouty swelling in great toe joint, better warmth, motion.

Thall: toes numb.

Neck

Rhodo: pain in right side, stiff, worse morning; night wet, weather.

Phyt: stiff, worse morning, motion, cold damp.

Cimic: stiff, contraction, feeling in females, worse morning and cold.

Bell: after exposure to cold-after cold wet.

Rhus tox: wet-effects, worse at rest.

Agust: stiff, cervical vertebrae involved.

Cereus: pain involving back, arms and fingers.

Note: Homoeopathic medicines for such problems should be started in low potencies like 6 or 30 - three to four drops three times a day for a week and if there is no response then you can take the selected medicines in 200 potency-four drops once in a week in early morning. If there is no response then please consult an experienced and qualified homoeopathic physician.

• • •

32

Headache–Homoeopathic Treatment

Homoeopathic medicines work on symptoms similarity. You can find a suitable remedy according to your symptoms.

Headache from Spine or Nape of Neck Goes Over Head

Sang. Can. 200–With flushes of heat and distended veins, of throbbing and lancinating nature, often begins in nape of neck or occiput and having come over head settles over eyes specially right side (Sit), wheezing in ears, nausea and vomiting; < morning till evening, in the noon; > in open air, sleep, lying down, copious urination, vomiting, pressing head with hands, rest and quietness.

Strontia C. 30–With vertigo and flushes of heat on face of throbbing and pulsating nature, begins in nape of neck and spreads over head to eyes or upper jaw, increases and decreases gradually nausea, < morning, evening, cold, lying with low; > wrapping head warmly, in the sun.

Silicea 200-With sweaty head, of sharp, tearing nature, begins in spine and spreads over head settling over eyes specially right eye, scalp sore, and sensitive to touch, sometimes nausea and vomiting, < by physical and mental exertion, jarring, motion, open air; > covering the head warmly, copious urination.

Phos. Ac. 200-With weight on vertex caused by strain or study, grief or disappointed love ; often begins in nape of neck and spreads upward < least motion, morning, music, exertion;> lying down.

Menyan. 200-With pressure and weight on vertex, sometimes begins in nape of neck and spreads over head; hands and feet cold. < on ascending stairs, one side, after eating. jarring;> by hard pressure by hands, stooping, sitting.

Iris. V. 30-With throbling and shooting, of bilious and periodical nature, begins in nape of neck and having spread over head settles in forehead, extending to right temple and dental nerves; often preceded by blurred vision which continues during pain, < cold air, coughing, motion, rest, lying down, night, right side; > open air, continued slow motion.

Spigelia 30-With protruding and squeezed feeling in left eye, sometimes begins in back of head and settles over left eye, increases and decreases with the sun, < in day only, jarring, stooping, straining at stool, morning till noon, night; > cold, rest, pressure.

Gelsemium 200-With feeling of a band around head and heavy eyelids with desire to keep them closed, begins in cervical spine or occiput and sometimes extending to temples, ears, wing of nose and even chin, of throbbing, hammering nature, thick speech and preceded by blurred vision and followed by frequent and copius urination, < tobacco smoking, heat of sun; > lying down, rest, sleep, pressure, urination head on raised pillow.

Cocc I. 200-With vertigo and bandage feelings, begins in occiput and spreads to nape of neck or spine, thought or smell of food us numb and empty feeling, shutting and opening sensation, eyes protruding specially in left side, < eating, jars> drinking, lying on back of head, cold and open air, sitting, after sleep, coffee, tobacco> in carriage; > indoors, rest, warmth, quietness.

Lac. C. 30 - From occiput to forehead, changes sides, nausea-vomiting, relaxation alternating with contraction.

Sec. C. 200 -Rising from back of head, dark bleeding from nose, pale face> by cold.

Headache from Forehead Goes Upward

Lac. D. 200- With blurred vision and obstinate constipation of throbbing nature, begins in forehead and spreads upward to occiput nausea, vomiting, copious urine, < light, motion, morning, during menses; > pressure and bandaging head tightly.

Oreod. 30-Begins in orbit and spreads through brain to the base of occiput sometimes to scapula or the spine or the ears, < 1. side, light; > closing eyes, silence and rest; constant aching in cervico-occipital region.

Pic. Ac. 30 - Begins in forehead and spreads over head to occiput, extending to neck or spine, < stooping, motion and mental exertion; > pressure bandaging tightly, open air.

Phytolacca 200 - With syphilitic taint, spreads upward, < in damp weather, > rest.

Naja. 200-With anxiety at heart (Calc. Ars., Cact), in left temple and teft orbital region, spreading upward to occiput, vomiting, < walking in the open air.

Nat. Mur. 200-With tendency to take cold and compressed feeling, sometimes begins in root of nose spreading upward to forehead, of throbbing, bursting, stitching and hammering nature; sometimes increases and decreases with the sun, eyes feel protruding nausea, vomiting; < on walking in the morning, mental exertion (reading, writing, etc.), cold air, coughing and sneezing, looking fixedly; > sitting, lying quietly with raised head, sleep, perspiration, open air.

Bufo. 200 - With flushes of heat, weight and pressure on vertex, wave of heat rising from solar plexus to the top of head in hysteric or epileptic patients, < light, > nose-bleed.

Ruta G. 6 - Of pulsating and pressing nature, sometimes begins in temporal regions and spreads to occiput, sometimes nail-driven feeling in head; < slightest eye-strain - reading, sewing, writing.

Tuber. 200 - In schoolgirls or tubercular patients or chronic headache on the verge of maniacal state, sometimes begins in r. eye and spreads to occiput, bandage feeling. < mental exertion.

Bryonia 30 - With constipation, thirst for large quantities of cold water, great dryness; sometimes begins in forehead and spreads over head to occiput; < motion, moving of eye balls, stooping, eating, right side, in the morning, > rest, lying quietly, nose-bleed.

Onos. 30 - Occipito-frontal headache often on I. side, in temples, often on I. side and in morning on waking; blurred vision.

Pulsatilla 30 - With dryness without thirst, with desire for open air, of erratic or shifting nature, enlargement of veins sometimes stitching extending to face and teeth; temporal pain with lachrymation from the same sided eye, < evening and warmth; > open air, pressure, bandaging head tightly.

Ipecac 30 - With persistent nausea, with bruised or sore feeling in skull-bones, extends to teeth and root of tongue, > temporarily by vomiting.

Rhodium 200 - With tearful disposition, extends to eyes, ears, nose,teeth and sometimes shoulders and arms. Pain sometimes extends to shoulders or arms.

Stell 2x - With sleeplessness and eye-protruding feeling extends to temples and back of head, shifting pains throughout the body, < morning and motion, r. or I. side.

Ferr. Met. 30- With flushes of heat in face, vertigo and anaemia, of hammering, pulsating and throbbing nature; extends to teeth,veins of head swollen, scalp sore and painful, aversion to eating and drinking, cold extremities, <I. side, after menses, after mid-night, lying down, > walking slowly, open air, pressure with hands.

Arg. Nit. 200-With feeling of fullness, heaviness, and enlargement, vertigo and buzzing in ears attack often ends in unconsciousness and bilious vomiting; pain extends to the corresponding eye; pain increases and decreases rapidly ; < often L. side, mental labour or emotion, dancing, > open air, pressure, bandaging head tightly.

Ptelea 30 - With red face and sore feeling on scalp, accompanied by hepatic disorders, sometimes extends to the root of nose and temples, < motion and night.

Note :- Drs. hold high opinion about Ptelea for frontal headache when other remedies fail.

Menthol 200 - Pain descends, to eye- balls, particularly L. eye, < option.

Chionanth 30 - Frontal with gastro hepatic disorders, extends to temples, root of nose and over eyes, sometimes nausea, vomiting, < stooping and motion, jar.

Euon 30-With constipation and albuminous urine, with increased acidity, pain extends to eye-brows turning to backside, < r. or L side. evening, > pressure.

Chin. Sulph 200 - With vertigo and distension of veins about head and neck, of pressing, tearing, throbbing and pulsating nature, extends to temples, < L. side, noon, morning till noon.

Note :- To be considered in malarial attacks.

Senecio Aur. Q. - With feeling of fullness and sneezing, extends over 1. eye and through I. temple, < after-noon.

Cimicifuga 30 - With uterine trouble of shooting lancinating and throbbing nature, extends to in-and-over eyes, sometimes to shoulders and spine; feels shutting and opening in scalp, feels as if top of head will fly away < evening, afternoon, indoors, during menses, > lying down, open air, bending the head forward.

Sepia 30 - With uterine troubles, sensation of weight on vertex, of pressing, boring and throbbing nature, extends to L. eye and L. temple; terrible forenoon to night; indoors, motion, stooping, jarring, evening, turning eyes; sitting, > Rest, external pressure, closing eyes, after sleep, in darkness.

Zinc Valero 30 - With uterine or ovarian trouble, hiccup sleeplessness, of piercing and stabbing nature, extends to spine, often in hysterical females.

Valer 200 - With cold feeling, of sticking, jerking, drawing, pressing and stupefying nature extends to the orbits, < evening, during rest, open air, > motion, indoors, change of position.

Menthol. - Frontal headache radiating to eye-balls and over frontal sinus with feeling of numbness and coldness in nose, deafness. < L. side.

Miscellaneous Headaches

Bell. 200 - With throbbing of carotids and flushed face during cold, coryza and fever of any kind, sometimes in r. side only, < noise, jar, light, cold, evening and bending head forward> closing eyes, pressure, wrapping.

Scutell- Frontal headache r. sided with aching to eyeballs as if pressed outwards and, < rest and night.

Oreod-Cervico occipital headache, nausea vomiting, colic,> in perfect quiet condition.

Glon. 30 - With flushed face and eye ball protruding-feeling, of throbbing and pulsating nature sometimes it is felt throughout the body, sometimes increases and decreases with the sun, < heat, motion, jar, bending head backward; > open air, fanning, uncovering, pressure, bandaging head tightly.

Cact. 30 - With a feeling of bandage about head, sensation, of weight on vertex, of throbbing and pulsating nature, distended blood-vessels, returns at the same time < r. side> eating, > pressure.

Kali C. 200- With lumbago and dryness of hair, of sticking nature particularly in temples, yawning one sided, < cold, open air, stooping, after midnight, morning; < raising the head.

Kali Bic. 30 - With sore feeling on the scalp, feeling of fulness which extends to the root of nose and angle of eye, one sided, preceded by blurred vision, which is > when headache increases, < morning till noon, on waking in the morning.

Cann. Ind. 200 - With talkativeness and forgetfulness, of throbbing nature with shutting and opening feeling in brain shocks in brain with shaking of head, heavy load feeling on head sometimes feeling as if cold water dropping on head, time and space seem long.

Melif 30 - With flushed face, blood-shot eyes and feeling of fulness all over head, of bursting and throbbing nature, retching and vomiting, sexual irritation < 9 A. M. till noon, afternoon, > copious urination, nose-bleed, menstrual flow, open air.

Nux Vom. 200 - With gastric derangement and feeling of chilliness, of bursting or tearing nature, retching with aversion to food, sometimes feels as if nail were driven in, < morning cold, eating, > rest and warm room (should be taken at bed time).

Paul S.-Headache after tea, coffee or liquor.

Ignatia 200-With tearful disposition as a result of grief, of tearing and sticking nature, feels as if a nail were driven in, <from eye-strain and mental exertion, strong odour, liquor, stooping> changing position, lying on back and painful side.

Coffea - 200 - With nervous exhaustion and sleeplessness, of tearing nature, feels as if a nail were driven in. < after sleep, eating, morning, open air, > sitting quietly, in room.

Thuja 30 - Often with sycotic history, one sided, feels as if a nail were driven in, particularly in r. temple and root of nose,

< morning, evening, motion, > open air, uncovering the head, perspiration, looking upward, bending head backward.

Agar. M. 200-With desire to cover head warmly, pulsating and twitching in facial muscles, feels as if a nail were driven in or as if icy needles were piercing into head sometimes the trouble extends to the root of nose, < cold air, standing.

Anac. 30 - With sexual irritation and irritability of mind, feels, as if a plug or nail were driven in < from exertion and excitement, > by eating.

Tarent. 200 - With formication and restlessness, feels as if needles were piercing into brain, < touch, strong light, > rubbing.

Ran B. 200 - With sleepiness, exhaustion and sense of enlargement of head, of bursting and pressing nature, < from change of temperature either from cold to warm or from warm to cold.

China 30-(10 to 15 drops at a time), with flushed face of patients worn out from loss of animal fluids, of bursting and throbbing nature, pulsation in carotids, < lying or sitting; > walking or standing.

Psor. 200-With increased appetite during attack and tendency to catch cold, of hammering, boring, pulsating and pressing nature, bandage feeling around head, < change of weather, cold winds, stooping, moving the eyes, fast walking, > eating, wrapping the head.

Merc. I Rub200 - With pain in bones of face, <night.

Aloes 30 - With heaviness in eyes compelling one to close them in those suffering from uterine or haemarhoidal trouble, headache alternates with lumbago < after stool on every foot-step < from cold applications.

Stict. P. 30- With pressure and fullness in forehead and at the root of nose, heat and soreness in eye-balls feels sometimes floating in the air < change of temperature, > discharges.

Zinc Met. 200 - With fidgetiness in legs and confused dullness in mind after suppressed discharges or eruptions, of pressing , tearing, stupefying and drawing nature, < in sides, > by discharges and open air.

Plat. 30 - With numb feeling here and there, creeping and cold sensation, changeable temperament - hot and cool, gay and grief alternately, pain increases and decreases gradually < evening in room, at rest, > rubbing and open air.

Mag. Mur. 30 - With roaring and numb feeling, sweating of head, constipation with accumulation of water in mouth, milk disagrees, of griping, squeezing and bursting nature; < morning, open air, wrapping head warmly, pressure with hands.

Sulphur 30 - With feeling of burning heat buzzing and roaring > heaviness and fullness, great heat in palms and soles, <of burning and pressing and pulsating nature, -< noon, evening, night, > open air, external pressure.

Asclep. Syr. lx- With obstinate constipation and copious urination, with increased specific gravity, feels as if a pointed instrument is pierced through one temple to the other, increased urine and perspiration follow headache.

Scutel. Lat. 6 - (5 drops a dose) - Frontal and at base of brain with dreams and frequent urination, aching in eye-balls, "feels as if eyes are protruding <right side, noise, odour, light> night, sleep.

All. Cepa 30 - With appearance of menses, < evening, warm room, > open air, when menses flow.

Viola Od. 30- With vertigo and burning in forehead.

Rhamnus 1x-With soreness and sensitiveness all over head, of bursting nature, in head, face and neck, constipation, <evening, bending forward, with every step.

Lach 200 - With septic states, bead and sensitiveness of the scalp, left sided, < on awaking.

Cycl. 200 - With flickering before eyes in anaemic -Women, menstrual disorder, < morning on waking, open air indoors.

Poly. Pin.-With pain in back, leg, ankle, < 10 a.m. to 3 p.m.

Lob.Inf. 30 - With perspilation, prostration and nausea, vomiting, from temple to temple, < afternoon to midnight.

Sabad. 6 - With dizziness and coryza; of pressing nature; often right sided, < from thinking intently or looking fixedly at one object, exertion or concentration > pressure and lying.

Carb. An. 30- With feeling as if head is going to tear into pieces, < night when lying down > sitting up and hold it tightly.

Crocus. S. 30- With black stringy menstrual flow, of throbbing, pulsating nature, < before, during and after flow.

Lit. T. 30. - With uterine and cardiac irritation, 'hot and wild feeling, > open air.

Tabac. 200 - With persistent nausea and violent vomiting, followed by sweats, < morning till noon and subsides by sun-set > open cold air.

Theriod. 30 - Pain deep in brain, < least sound and least motion of head.

Ant. C. 200- With milky white coated tongue, < from the heat of the sun.

Hyper. 6 - With feeling of soreness in eyes, feels as if lifted up high in the air, effects of fall.

Gauiacum 30- Of rheumatic character spreading to face and neck.

Note:- 200 potency is to be repeated after a week while

30 potency is to be taken 3-4 drops thrice a day.

• • •

33

Ayurvedic Treatment of Migraine

Migraine has become a common disorder owing to modern lifestyle.From the perspective of ayurveda, migraine headaches are due to a disorder in *tridosha* - the mind-body constitution. Although it is possible to get headaches from disorders in *vata*, *pitta*, or *kapha*, migraines frequently occur when systemic *pitta* moves into the cardiovascular system, circulates, and affects the blood vessels around the brain. The blood vessels dilate due to the hot, sharp quality of *pitta*. This, in turn, creates pressure on the nerves, resulting in migraines. *Pitta* disorders are characterized by the red complexion and eyes, light sensitivity, burning sensation, anger, irritability, and nose bleeds. So, the treatment involves following the recommendations for *pitta* pacifying foods, herbs and lifestyle.

Avoid hot, spicy foods, fermented foods, and sour or citrus fruits. A *pitta*-soothing diet is effective both for migraine relief and as a preventive measure.

Preventive Breakfast

If you are one of those individuals who get migraines at midday, which then subside later in the evening, there is a preventive approach available from ayurveda. It is simple, but effective.

First thing in the morning, take 1 ripe banana. Peel it, chop it into pieces, and add 1 teaspoon warm ghee, 1 teaspoon date sugar, and a pinch of cardamom on top. This is delicious, and it will help to reduce *pitta* and prevent a headache from arising.

Herbal Remedy

The following herbal compound is beneficial in managing migraine.

shatavari 5 parts
brahmi 4 parts
jatamamsi 3 parts
musta 3 parts

Prepare this mixture, and take 1/2 teaspoon twice a day, morning and evening, after breakfast and dinner, with a little lukewarm water. This formula is designed to pacify the aggravated *pitta* and help relieve migraine headaches.

Purgatives (such as aloe vera gel, rhubarb, and fennel), liver cleansers (such as bhamiamalaki and brahmi), sandalwood oil on the third eye, temples, heart, and under the nose, medicated oils or ghee, using gudachi, bala, and ashwagandha; fomentation, and saturating snuff are also advised.

Long-term healing includes chyavan prash, brahmi, and ashwagandha.

Other Treatments

Avoid Direct Sun

Because migraine headaches are predominantly a *pitta* disorder, they are affected by the hot sun. When the sun rises, its hot, sharp, penetrating rays increase *pitta* in the cardiovascular system and cause the dilation of the blood vessels in the brain, which results in the painful headaches. So avoid direct exposure to the sun. If you have to go out, use an umbrella or wear a hat or other protection from the sun.

Nature walks

Walks in the full moon and by water; and flower gardening reduce *Pitta* causes of migraines.

Soothing Nose Drops

Once a headache has developed, putting about 5 drops of warm brahmi ghee in each nostril will help relieve the pain.

Head Massage

Shiro dhara (hot oil head massage) is also beneficial.

Recommended Yoga Postures

Moon Salutation is especially good for migraines. Yoga postures such as the Hidden Lotus, Boat pose, Bow pose, Spinal Twist, Palm Tree pose, and Standing on the Toes are also good to combat migraines.

A Cooling Pranayama

Do a cooling breathing exercise such as shitali. To do it, curl your tongue into a tube. Inhale slowly through the curled tongue, swallow, and then exhale normally through the nose, keeping the mouth closed. You will feet the incoming air cool your saliva, your tongue, and the oral mucous membranes.

This breathing exercise will lower the body temperature, and make the saliva cool. It also helps to quench thirst, and improves digestion, absorption, and assimilation.

If you can't curl your tongue into a tube, an alternative way to perform shitali is with your teeth lightly clenched together and your tongue pressed up against the teeth. The air is then inhaled through the teeth.

Some people feel pain when cool air is drawn through the teeth; keeping your tongue against your teeth will provide warmth and prevent this discomfort.

A Healing Yawn

When you have a migraine, gently squeeze your earlobes, pulling the ear down, and do the act of yawning. This will relieve the pressure on the blood vessels and help to pacify the headache.

Avoid overexertion

Migraines from *Vata* Imbalance:

As mentioned migraines can also originate due to imbalance in *vata dosha*. The symptoms of *vata* imbalance are: anxiety, depression, dry skin, constipation, and extreme pain. The recommended treatment is: triphala as a purgative, jatamanshi, brahmi, and rest. Shiro dhara (hot oil head massage) is also recommended.

Migraines from *Kapha* Imbalance:

This condition is characterized by dull headache, heaviness, fatigue, nausea, white or clear phlegm, vomiting, and excess salivation. Respiratory disorders are often associated with these symptoms. The recommended treatment is: trikatu, brahmi, tulsi tea, inhaling eucalyptus oil, vomiting, exercise, nasal snuff of ginger or pepper. Shiro dhara (hot oil head massage) is also recommended.

Suvarna Sutashekhara

This is the most commonly prescribed Ayurvedic drug for treating migraine. It is not just a preventive but also a curative means.

Ingredients: Many items are used to prepare this medication. These elements are borax and sulphur in the 'bhasma' form, sulphur, copper, gold and mercury.

Moreover, 10 medicinal plants and drugs (extracted from animal sources) are added to the mixture.

Besides, two other strong drugs (which are poisonous in their raw forms) – Dhatura and Vatsanabha – are processed to make them not only potent but also pure. After processing, these two drugs are made free from having any side effects on a patient.

All of these are mixed in definite ratios. To this mixture is added Bhringaraja juice.

Dose: It is given in the dose of 125 milligram twice daily. The medication is to be taken with milk.

Godanti Bhasma

This is a rather inexpensive but effective Ayurvedic medication for patients suffering from migraine.

Dose: It is given in the dose of one gram thrice daily. The medication is to be taken with honey.

Shadbindu Taila

This Ayurvedic medicated oil is quite effective in treating migraine. This medication irritates the nasal mucous membrane. However, it effects instant relief.

Ingredient: This drug is to be taken with mustard oil.

Dose : Only six drops are to be taken in each nostril daily and till the symptoms persist.

Anu Taila

Proper use of this oil brings about instant relief to acute and chronic migraine instances.

This medicated oil needs to be inhaled deeply to induce forced sneezing. It removes the nasal blockages from the sinuses and their passages. The nerves in the nasal routes are soothed.

Even as the mental strain is removed, the heaviness in the head is also relieved. The patient will be able to sleep soundly. Above all, there are no side effects.

Ingredients : It is prepared from 26 medicinal plants. The definite proportions of these plants are then boiled in goat's milk and gingelly oil.

Dose : *One needs to drop at least 15 drops of this oil in each nostril to induce sneezing.* This medicated oil needs to be inhaled at least thrice daily.

Panchakarma for Migraine and Headaches

Pre-purification therapies:Pre-purification therapies are the first ones applied to loosen the toxins, open up the circulation channels and get the body ready for discarding these wastes. These methods are highly relaxing for the body and mind.

The following pre-purification methods are usually adopted for treating Migraines and Headaches.

Sirodhara: In this process herbal oil, medicated milk, medicated butter milk etc., are poured on the forehead in a special method for about 45-50 minutes. Highly effective in providing both temporary and permanent relief from Migraines and Headaches. Ingredients used in Sirodhara include gooseberry, sandalwood.

Thakradhara :This treatment involves continuous pouring of medicated buttermilk on the forehead. It cools the head and gives immediate relief from headaches. It also has a soothing effect on the eyes. Amaltas, nut grass tuber and staff tree are the medicinal herbs used.

Thalam Special powder mixed with medicated oil is applied on head vertex and retained for 20 to 45 minutes. Medicinal herbs used are Sida plant Indian Penny worth and the Staff tree.

• • •

34

Home Treatment of Migraine

Wet a towel, squeeze it and keep it in the freezer for around 5 – 7 minutes. Now, take the frozen towel and keep it over your head and eyes. You will notice immediate relief from the severe pain. Another highly effective alternative is to opt for a good head/scalp massage. Lie down in a room that is dark and peaceful and without any environmental disturbances. Allow a massage expert to gently apply flowing strokes to your head and scalp to bring you relief from the pain. In the absence of a massage therapist, you may try massaging the head yourself. This can be done by massaging the scalp and head by rubbing the aching areas in gentle circular motions.

Aromatherapy has been found to be quite effective in relieving the painful symptoms of a migraine attack. In aromatherapy, the most regularly used essential oils used for providing relief from migraine attacks include lavender and peppermint. These essential oils are helpful in easing stress, tensions and migraines. Do bear in mind that not all individuals find relief from using aromatherapy. Ginger is one of the most effective solutions to ease pain caused during migraine attacks. It has a high content of anti inflammatory properties, which are beneficial in promoting blood circulation and relaxing the blood vessels. The consumption of fresh ginger or powdered ginger in a slightly cooked form can also prove to be advantageous in obtaining relief from pain caused due to migraine attack.

Always remember to drink lots of water. Keeping one's self well hydrated is believed to be one of the most effective home remedies for migraine attacks. There are many cases where headaches can begin due to severe dehydration and thus it is extremely critical to ensure that you drink sufficient amounts of water. Ideally, it is recommended that you drink about a litre of water daily.

Identify the reasons which are triggering your attacks. There are different triggers for different individuals. Some individuals are affected by a particular food whereas others are affected by excessive stress. Determining your specific triggers will help you in preventing migraine attacks in the future.

Once used to treat a variety of conditions, including headaches and fever, feverfew has been "rediscovered" by migraine sufferers, who are using the herb to blunt the sometimes crippling pain that accompanies their sudden and ill-understood attacks.

Scientists now know that feverfew contains chemicals that may prevent migraines. And the best news is that feverfew has few side effects. Continue to the next page to learn more about feverfew and migraine pain relief.

Some people get some relief by applying either a cold or warm compress to the effected area. Most people report that a cold compress works best, but if that is not effective, try a warm compress.

Acupressure is also one of the good home remedies for migraine headaches. Like acupuncture, it is a well-known alternative treatment for many medical problems that has been used for thousands of years. To get headache pain relief, squeeze the fleshy area between your thumb and forefinger for at least five minutes for one of the quick remedies for migraines. Many folks also can relieve migraine pain by gently rubbing [using small circular motions] the little indentations just in front of your ears.

• • •

35

Tips for Headaches

Try the following tips for your occasional headache pain. If your headaches are frequent or severe, be sure to discuss them with a medical professional.

Try—but don't overdo—pain pills. A dose of an over-the-counter (OTC) analgesic, such as aspirin, acetaminophen, or ibuprofen, is often enough to alleviate the occasional headache. But if you take more than two doses a day frequently or for more than four or five days in a row to relieve headache pain, contact your doctor. Taking pain relievers too often can actually worsen your headache pain. For a list of precautions to take when using over-the-counter analgesics.

Lie down. Lying down and closing your eyes for half an hour or more may be one of the best treatments for a bad headache. For some types of headaches, such as migraines, sleep is the only thing that seems to interrupt the pain cycle. Recognizing the early signs of a headache can keep the pain from getting out of control, since doctors say the sooner you get to bed or lie on a sofa, the sooner a headache will fade.

Don't let the sun shine in. Especially if your symptoms resemble those of a migraine (such as severe pain on one side of the head, nausea, blurred vision, and extreme sensitivity to light), resting in a darkened room may alleviate the pain, experts agree. Bright light may also cause headaches. Even staring at a glowing computer screen may be enough to trigger pain on the brain. Wearing tinted glasses or using other means to filter bright light and minimize glare may help prevent headaches.

Use a cold compress. A washcloth dipped in ice-cold water and placed over the eyes or an ice pack placed on the site of the pain are other good ways of relieving a headache. You might also see if your pharmacy sells special ice packs that surround the whole head (known as "headache hats") or frozen gel-packs that can be inserted into pillows. Whatever you use, keep in mind that speed is critical: Using ice as soon as possible after the onset of the headache will relieve the pain within 20 minutes for most people.

Try heat. If ice feels uncomfortable to you, or if it doesn't help your headache, try placing a warm washcloth over your eyes or on the site of the pain. Leave the compress on for half an hour, rewarming it as necessary.

Think pleasant thoughts. Many headaches are brought on or worsened by stress and tension. Learning to handle life's difficulties by tuning out unpleasant thoughts may keep the volume down on a bad headache. When you feel your body shifting into crisis mode after you have a serious disagreement with a spouse or coworker, for example—force yourself to think pleasant thoughts. Relaxing your mind will help you figure out a way to resolve the problem, which can help ward off headache-causing tension.

Check for tension. Along with the preceding tip, stop periodically during the day and check your body for tension. Are you clenching your jaw or wrinkling your brow? Are your hands balled-up into fists? If you discover these signs of tension, stop, relax, and take a deep breath or two (don't go beyond a couple of deep breaths, though, otherwise you may begin to hyperventilate). Occasional body checks like this could nip a headache in the bud.

Quit smoking. Smoking may bring on or worsen a headache, especially if you suffer from cluster headaches—extremely painful headaches that last from 5 to 20 minutes and come in groups.

Don't drink. Drinking more alcohol than you're used to often causes a notorious morning-after effect—a pounding headache. But even a single serving of some alcoholic beverages can trigger headaches, including the migraine and cluster varieties, in certain people. For example, dark alcoholic beverages such as red wines, sherry, brandy, scotch, vermouth, and beer contain large amounts of tyramine, an amino acid that can spark headaches in people who are sensitive to it. And some people appear to be sensitive to the histamine in beer and wine. So if you're struggling with headaches, abstaining may be your best choice.

Start a programme of regular exercise. Regular exercise helps release the physical and emotional tension that may lead to headaches. Walking, jogging, and other aerobic activities help boost the body's production of endorphins (natural pain-relieving substances).

Cut down on caffeine. The same chemical in coffee and tea that perks you up in the morning can also make your muscles tense and send your anxiety level through the roof. Consuming too much caffeine can also cause insomnia, which can trigger headaches. Another problem is that many people drink several cups of coffee a day during their work week but cut their consumption on Saturdays and Sundays. This pattern can lead to weekend caffeine-withdrawal headaches.

If caffeine is giving you a headache, wean yourself off the stimulating stuff by cutting your intake slowly. Start by eliminating the equivalent of one-half cup coffee per week until you are only drinking one cup of caffeinated coffee (or its equivalent) per day. One five-ounce cup of drip coffee contains about 150 milligrams of caffeine. A five-ounce cup of tea brewed for three to five minutes may contain 20 to 50 milligrams of caffeine. And cola drinks contain about 35 to 45 milligrams of caffeine per 12-ounce serving. Look out for stealth sources of caffeine, too, particularly in the OTC drugs in your medicine cabinet.

Fight the nausea first. Some headaches may be accompanied by nausea, which can make you feel even worse. What's more, the gastric juices produced by stomach upset may hinder the absorption of certain prescription and OTC analgesics, which may make these drugs less effective at relieving the pain of your headache. So by first taking care of the nausea, the pain of the headache may be easier to treat. Many patients find that drinking peach juice, apricot nectar, or flat cola helps alleviate nausea. OTC antinauseants such as Emetrol and Dramamine may also be useful.

Rise and retire at the same time every day. Oversleeping can create changes in body chemistry that set off migraines and other headaches. Going to bed and getting up at the same time every day—including weekends—keeps your body in a stable rhythm.

Keep a headache diary. If you get frequent headaches, try to tease out the factors that seem to be responsible. Get a notebook and keep track of your headaches. Rate each one on a scale of 0 to 3, starting with no headache (a score of 0) and moving up in intensity to mild headache (a score of 1), moderate to severe headache (a score of 2), and incapacitating headache (a score of 3). Record details about potential headache triggers. Were you under an unusual amount of stress? What did you eat? If you're a woman, did you have your period? Did you use medications that contain hormones, such as oral contraceptives? Now look for patterns by connecting days when you had bad headaches with these factors. This information may help you avoid triggers and can also help your physician devise a better treatment plan.

• • •

36

Water Wonder

An old Japanese gentleman who enjoyed perfect health, was once met by a curious professor. When asked about the secret of his robust constitution, the old man explained that it was thanks to the Water Wonder. He went on to tell in detail about his sickly youth, when he was bed-ridden, with impaired intestines, for almost ten years. When all the modes of treatment failed to bring even partial relief from his sickness, he was told it was impossible to get a cure. One of the physicians who treated him, however, suggested a specific type of water treatment as a last resort.

The effect of the treatment was felt on the very first day and his appetite was restored, his digestion improved and within a few days he was cured of his chronic disease. It might have been a coincidence that the treatment he underwent all those years showed results only after this simple water treatment. So impressed with this treatment was he, that he tried it on the members of his family who were suffering from various illnesses ranging from brain fever to obesity and achieved positive results.

What is the Water Magic ?

The process is as follows:- Go to sleep three hours after a fairly early dinner around 7.00 p.m. Strictly do not eat or drink anything after that. Rise early from bed the next morning, do not wash your face and mouth as you do normally. Sit comfortably and drink six glasses of pure water at a stretch. If you find difficulty in doing so, pause a while after two or three glasses and continue. For the next 20 minutes walk briskly or do some exercise. Within twenty minutes to half an hour, urge to pass urine will be great and you will pass urine in large quantities quite frequently. Some may bring out the morbid waste through vomiting. Passing of stools will be easy and complete. It will facilitate the expulsion of the accumulated waste matter very effectively and leave you fresh.

• • •

Other Books on Health

1.	Ayurveda for All (New)	150/-
2.	A Guide to Migraine, Arthritis, Cervical Spondylosis and Backache (New)	125/-
3.	Body and Beauty Care (New)	125/-
4.	Yoga for All (New)	250/-
5.	Child Care and Nutrition (New)	95/-
6.	Naturopathy Modern Way of Life (New)	125/-
7.	A Guide to Your Pregnancy (New)	150/-
8.	First Aid (How to Handle an Accident)	125/-
9.	Acupressure in Daily Life	125/-
10.	Complete Book of Yoga	150/-
11.	Look Younger at any Age	125/-
12.	HIV/AIDS-Transmission, Prevention	110/-
13.	Diabetics and Diet	110/-
14.	Increase your Height & Loose your Weight	125/-
15.	Make Fitness A Way of Life	195/-
16.	Common Problems of Children	150/-
17.	Handbook of Nutrition and Dietetics	250/-
18.	A Guide to Massage Therapy	125/-
19.	A Guide to Family Medicine	150/-
20.	A Guide to Digestive Disorders	125/-
21.	Complete Book of Child Care	150/-
22.	A Guide to Homoeopathy	125/-
23.	Life Begins at 40	125/-
24.	Alternative Therapies	125/-